100 Questions & Answers About Myelodysplastic Syndromes

Jason Gotlib, MD, MS
Assistant Professor of Medicine
Division of Hematology
Stanford Cancer Center
Stanford, CA

Lenn Fechter, RN, BSN
Division of Hematology
Stanford Cancer Center
Stanford, CA

JONES AND BARTLETT PUBLISHERS
Sudbury, Massachusetts
BOSTON   TORONTO   LONDON   SINGAPORE

World Headquarters

Jones and Bartlett Publishers
40 Tall Pine Drive
Sudbury, MA 01776
978-443-5000
info@jbpub.com
www.jbpub.com

Jones and Bartlett Publishers
Canada
6339 Ormindale Way
Mississauga, Ontario L5V 1J2
Canada

Jones and Bartlett Publishers
International
Barb House, Barb Mews
London W6 7PA
United Kingdom

Jones and Bartlett's books and products are available through most bookstores and online booksellers. To contact Jones and Bartlett Publishers directly, call 800-832-0034, fax 978-443-8000, or visit our website www.jbpub.com.

Substantial discounts on bulk quantities of Jones and Bartlett's publications are available to corporations, professional associations, and other qualified organizations. For details and specific discount information, contact the special sales department at Jones and Bartlett via the above contact information or send an email to specialsales@jbpub.com.

The authors, editor, and publisher have made every effort to provide accurate information. However, they are not responsible for errors, omissions, or for any outcomes related to the use of the contents of this book and take no responsibility for the use of the products and procedures described. Treatments and side effects described in this book may not be applicable to all people; likewise, some people may require a dose or experience a side effect that is not described herein. Drugs and medical devices are discussed that may have limited availability controlled by the Food and Drug Administration (FDA) for use only in a research study or clinical trial. Research, clinical practice, and government regulations often change the accepted standard in this field. When consideration is being given to use of any drug in the clinical setting, the health care provider or reader is responsible for determining FDA status of the drug, reading the package insert, and reviewing prescribing information for the most up-to-date recommendations on dose, precautions, and contraindications, and determining the appropriate usage for the product. This is especially important in the case of drugs that are new or seldom used.

Production Credits
Executive Publisher: Christopher Davis
Associate Editor: Kathy Richardson
Editorial Assistant: Jessica Acox
Production Director: Amy Rose
Senior Production Editor: Jenny Bagdigian
Associate Marketing Manager: Rebecca Wasley
Director of Special Markets: Eileen Ward
Manufacturing Buyer: Therese Connell
Cover Design: Jonathon Ayotte
Cover Images: Middle-aged man © Rex Rover/Shutterstock, Inc.; elderly couple © iofoto/Shutterstock, Inc.; elderly woman © Elena Ray/Shutterstock, Inc.
Printing and Binding: Malloy, Inc.
Cover Printing: Malloy, Inc.

Library of Congress Cataloging-in-Publication Data
Gotlib, Jason R.
    100 Q&A about myelodysplastic syndromes / Jason R. Gotlib, Lenora Fechter.
      p. cm.
    Includes index.
    ISBN-13: 978-0-7637-5333-7
    ISBN-10: 0-7637-5333-5
    1. Myelodysplastic syndromes—Popular works. 2. Myelodysplastic syndromes—Miscellanea. I. Fechter, Lenora. II. Title. III. Title: One hundred Q&A about myelodysplastic syndromes. IV. Title: 100 questions and answers about myelodysplastic syndromes.
    RC645.73.G68 2007
    616.4'1—dc22
                                      2007046892

6048

Printed in the United States of America
11 10 09 08 07   10 9 8 7 6 5 4 3 2 1

To Our Patients and Their Families

Contents

Part One: The Basics   1

Questions 1–11 provide background on how blood cells are formed and what happens in MDS, including:

- What is myelodysplastic syndromes (MDS)?
- How common is MDS?
- What causes MDS?

Part Two: Diagnosis, Classification, and Prognosis   17

Questions 12–20 describe the steps leading to a diagnosis of MDS, such as:

- Is MDS one disease or a syndrome of similarly related diseases?
- How is MDS diagnosed?
- What is involved in a bone marrow biopsy? What information does the biopsy provide?

Part Three: Symptoms and Treatment Options   37

Questions 21–29 discuss common symptoms of MDS and the treatment options available, including:

- How is response evaluated in MDS?
- What are the most common presenting symptoms in MDS?
- What factors are weighed when evaluating specific treatment options for MDS?

Part Four: Treatment, Supportive Care, and Side Effects   51

Questions 30–68 describe specific treatments, supportive care, and side effects with such questions as:

- What is the difference between treatment and supportive care?
- When do I need a red blood cell transfusion?
- What does it mean if I develop antibodies to red blood cells or platelet transfusions?
- Is there a role for chemotherapy in the treatment of MDS?

In 1994, a group of approximately 80 hematologists and oncologists met in Chicago, Illinois, at the Third International Symposium on Myelodysplastic Syndromes (MDS). No effective established therapies were available at that time for patients with MDS. The group recognized that the confusing French–American–British system of classification of MDS offered only modest prognostic information to this heterogeneous patient population. Although researchers presented results of several clinical trials at the meeting, each trial used a different 'homespun' set of criteria to evaluate response to the new treatments. Most patients in the early 1990s received supportive care, with transfusions of blood products and antibiotics when needed. Physicians often did not go out of their way to diagnose MDS in anemic patients because no effective treatments were available. Hematologists historically resisted calling MDS "leukemia" or "cancer," and as a result the national cancer registries did not collect any information on MDS cases. Thus none of the investigators could estimate how common this problem was.

In 2007, the same organization met in Florence, Italy. The U.S. Food and Drug Administration had recently approved three effective drugs for the treatment of MDS, as well as a new drug for the treatment of iron over-accumulation. The World Health Organization had reclassified MDS and the related disorder chronic myelomonocytic leukemia in a still somewhat controversial system that recognizes subgroups of MDS with more specific biological behavior and prognoses. In 1997, investigators had published results of a collaboration begun at the Chicago meeting, which defined a clinically useful prognostic score—the International Prognostic Scoring System (IPSS). Since 2000, clinical researchers have used a standard set of criteria to evaluate new drugs, so that the results of different clinical trials could be better compared. The national cancer registries recognized and subsequently tracked the frequency of MDS as a malignant disease in 2002.

Preliminary data suggest that 5-azacitidine might in fact improve survival in patients with high-risk MDS in addition to improving blood counts. Several new drugs, drug combinations, and new approaches to stem cell transplantation show great promise for MDS patients.

With all the positive developments in MDS, the disease(s) continues to be heterogeneous, and the field can be complicated for patients. Newly diagnosed patients who previously knew nothing about blood cells need to become educated about the nuances of red cells, hemoglobin, hematocrit, different types of white blood cells, blast cells, transfusions, and the significance of acute leukemias. In addition, patients need to be able to understand the details of their particular disorder, its prognosis, and the likelihood of various therapies to affect their survival and quality of life.

Many patients find these tasks daunting. Physicians are often too busy to spend adequate time educating the patient about these complex disorders. Although several helpful resources exist—particularly the publications and websites of the MDS Foundation, the Aplastic Anemia and MDS International Foundation, and the Physician's Data Query from the National Cancer Institute—*100 Questions & Answers About Myelodysplastic Syndromes* represents a wonderful new "one-stop-shopping" go-to guide for MDS patients. In clear, patient-friendly language, Dr. Jason Gotlib and registered nurse Lenn Fechter walk patients through the complex definitions, classifications, prognostic factors, and treatments for MDS, as well as basics on how to choose a hematologist, prepare advanced directives, and approach clinical trials. The text is thoughtful, accurate, and balanced as it presents the current state of the science. It is a resource that I will certainly direct my patients to as they begin their journey through this complex arena—a journey that at last has a great deal of light shining through the portico.

Steven D. Gore, MD
Associate Professor of Oncology
The Sidney Kimmel Comprehensive Cancer Center
Johns Hopkins Medicine

Let's start with the name: "Myelodysplastic Syndromes." It's an enigmatic medical term that when first uttered by the doctor is often met with patient bewilderment. A typical response is, "Myelo...what?" With approximately 10,000 to 15,000 new cases diagnosed yearly in the United States, MDS is considered a relatively uncommon illness. It is partly for this reason that it also lacks the media exposure and familiarity associated with more identifiable blood cancers or solid tumors, such as acute leukemia and lung, colon, breast, and prostate cancers. Despite these caveats, MDS is one of the most common reasons for referral of older individuals to a hematologist, usually because of unexplained anemia or other low blood counts.

The purpose of this book is to remove the veil of obscurity and confusion that surrounds the diagnosis, biology, classification, and treatment of MDS. Making a disease more accessible and understandable to patients and their families is a vital mission of the doctor. Achieving this goal is sometimes handicapped, however, by the pressured time of the office visit, and the failure to translate 'medical-speak' into familiar language. Doctors who treat MDS may use terms loosely and interchangeably to describe it: "bone marrow cancer," "bone marrow failure," "chronic anemia," or "pre-leukemia." None of these terms necessarily describes MDS accurately or completely in a particular individual.

The complex biology of MDS and its variable presentation and prognosis have certainly contributed to the mystification of MDS. For example, how is it possible that for two 60-year-old patients with MDS, one may require no treatment and one may require a high-intensity therapy? Factors such as age, co-existing medical illnesses and functional capacity, stage of MDS, and personal goals of care all intersect in the decision to pursue treatment and the specific options available. It is also important for health care providers to approach MDS not only as a disease, but more broadly as an illness whose impact extends beyond physical functioning of the patient to psychosocial, spiritual, and economic domains of life.

Although your hematologist should be the primary source of information as it relates to your MDS, the emergence of the Internet has proven to be a rich source of information as well. There is, however, notorious inconsistency in the quality and accuracy of websites. It can be difficult to filter extraneous information or to gauge what data relates to a patient's specific MDS subtype. Uncensored information and online patient testimonials can also provoke some patients to take unproven and anxiety-filled detours off of this information highway. With *100 Questions & Answers About Myelodysplastic Syndromes,* our aim was to create a comprehensive companion for MDS patients as they navigate their illness, and to provide a listing of reliable resources for individuals seeking additional information. This book arrives at a time in which there has been increasing optimism amongst investigators who study and treat MDS. This promising outlook reflects the explosion in basic research and clinical advances in the disease over the last 10 years, culminating in the recent FDA approval of the first drugs to treat MDS since the disease was recognized in the 1950s.

Jason Gotlib, MD, MS
Lenn Fechter, RN, BSN

PART ONE

The Basics

What is myelodysplastic syndromes (MDS)?

How common is MDS?

What causes MDS?

More . . .

1. What is myelodysplastic syndromes (MDS)?

In the human body, blood is composed of three general types of cells: **red blood cells, white blood cells,** and **platelets**. These cells are manufactured in the **bone marrow**, which is the soft tissue in the center of the bones. The term **myelodysplastic syndromes**, or **MDS,** refers to a group of similar blood disorders. Each of these disorders is characterized by two common features: first, the bone marrow is unable to provide enough normal blood cells into the **circulation,** and second, in all MDS subtypes, the marrow produces blood cells that are misshapen. The abnormal appearance of these cells (referred to as dysplasia; see Question 4) can be seen when a blood or bone marrow sample is viewed under the microscope. However, MDS is considered a syndrome rather than a distinct disease because there are many different ways in which these problems can appear. In some patients, MDS causes a decline in red blood cells that may be stable for many years, but no other blood cells are affected. In others, both red and white blood cell counts are low, which can make a person more likely to get infections—or the patient might have a low platelet count instead, which can cause him or her to bleed and bruise more easily than normal. A number of different combinations of low red, white, and platelet counts are possible. In some cases, the changes within the bone marrow of MDS patients can lead to acute myelogenous leukemia, a cancer of the white blood cells (see Question 8).

2. How common is MDS?

It is difficult to say exactly how many people currently have MDS because it has not been reported for very long to the United States Cancer Surveillance Pro-

Red blood cells

blood cells that transport oxygen from the lungs to the tissues.

White blood cells

blood cells that fight infection, attack disease, mediate allergic responses, and heal damage to the body.

Platelets

blood cells that are important for clotting.

Bone marrow

the central tissue of bones in which blood cells are formed.

Circulation

the complete system of blood vessels that transports fluids, nutrients, and wastes in the body.

gram, which consists of a national database named **Surveillance, Epidemiology, and End Results (SEER)**. Data on MDS were collected for the first time by SEER in 2001. The SEER data were assembled from 17 regions in the United States, representing 76 million persons; the first analysis of this data set was published in March 2007.[1] The researchers found that 10,300 new cases of MDS were diagnosed in 2003, and that more men were diagnosed with MDS than women (4.5 versus 2.7 cases per 100,000 persons per year). They also found that MDS was most common in white individuals, and least common in Native Americans, Inuits, and Asian/Pacific Islanders. The SEER database is considered the most authoritative program for reporting disease **incidence** in the United States; however, because many physicians are not yet aware of the need to report MDS, there may still be some under-reporting of the syndrome. Although MDS is relatively common for a blood disorder, the absolute number of cases is considerably fewer than more common cancers such as breast, lung, colon, or prostate cancer. New cases of each of these diseases are reported annually in the range of tens of thousands of cases, up to as many as 200,000 cases each year.

Surveillance, Epidemiology, and End Results (SEER)

a national database of cancer diagnoses that calculates the relative frequency of different cancers in the American population.

Incidence

a measure of new cases of a disease in a specific population during a particular time frame.

3. What is the age range of patients affected by MDS?

The risk of developing MDS increases with age for both men and women. Recent statistics from SEER indicate that 86% of MDS cases were diagnosed in patients older than 60, and the average age at diagnosis

---

[1]Ma X, Does M, Raza A, Mayne ST. Myelodysplastic syndromes: incidence and survival in the United States. *Cancer* 2007; 109:1536–1542.

The Basics

was 76 years.[2] Although MDS is relatively uncommon under the age of 50, rare cases of MDS have been diagnosed in children and in adults 20 to 30 years of age.

4. What does "dysplasia" mean?

It is important for your doctor to rule out other causes of dysplasia and low blood counts before diagnosing MDS.

Dysplasia is a medical term that refers to the abnormal appearance of cells when viewed under a microscope. Dysplasia of blood cells is seen in the blood or bone marrow of patients with MDS. Physicians and pathologists who see large numbers of patients with MDS will be able to recognize the subtle signs of dysplasia in the blood or bone marrow of patients with very early signs of MDS, such as mild anemia.

Dysplasia of red blood cells has been one traditional requirement to make a diagnosis of MDS. Red blood cells are normally round disks that curve inward on the flat sides (Figure 1). Enlarged or oval-shaped red blood cells as shown in the figure are an example of dysplastic red cells. White blood cells and/or platelets may also be dysplastic in the blood or bone marrow of

---

[2]Ibid.

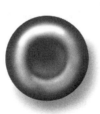 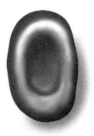

Normal red blood cell   Macro-ovalocytic red blood cell

Figure 1

MDS patients. A dysplastic white blood cell may have an abnormally shaped **nucleus** or contain fewer **granules** in the cells (a condition called **hypogranularity**). Platelets may also exhibit different types of dysplasia, including hypogranularity and large or bizarre shapes (Figure 2).

Dysplasia of blood cells doesn't only happen with MDS; it can be also be seen in completely unrelated conditions, including significant alcohol intake, HIV infection, **nutritional deficiencies** (for example, deficiencies of vitamin B_{12}, folate, or copper), and exposure to **toxins**. These conditions also may cause low blood counts. Therefore, it is important for your treating doctor to rule out these other conditions, particularly since some of these other causes are much easier to treat. For example, we have consulted on patients who were told they had MDS when they actually had pernicious anemia, an autoimmune disease that leads to decreased absorption of vitamin B12, and ultimately, to changes in blood cells that can resemble MDS. Alcohol use is another very common factor that can cause blood cell changes similar to those seen in MDS, and someone with MDS-like dysplasia of the blood cells must stop using alcohol altogether for at least 6 months in order to rule out alcohol as the cause

Nucleus

the structure within a cell that contains the cell's genetic material.

Granule

a small particle within a cell that can be seen by light or electron microscopy; contains stored material.

Hypogranularity

a condition in which cells contain fewer granules than normal.

Nutritional deficiency

a condition in which intake of an important mineral, vitamin, or nutrient is insufficient for good health.

Toxins

a poison; a substance that damages or harms a living organism or its cells.

The Basics

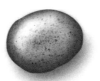

Normal-sized platelet　　　Large, hypogranular platelet

Figure 2

of the condition. If the dysplasia and low blood counts don't improve after six months of abstinence from alcohol, then a diagnosis of MDS may be more likely.

5. Will I give MDS to my children? Is MDS hereditary?

MDS is most often an acquired bone marrow disorder that is usually diagnosed in older individuals. Inherited (familial) cases of MDS are rare, and individuals with familial MDS are usually diagnosed with their disease at an earlier age (that is, before the age of 50). Therefore, it is extremely unlikely that MDS can be passed to one's children unless there is an established history of MDS, or a similar blood disorder such as acute myelogenous leukemia (AML), already diagnosed in more than one closely-related family member—a parent, aunt, uncle, or sibling.

6. What causes MDS?

In the overwhelming majority of cases, there is no clear reason why a particular individual might develop MDS. The bone marrow failure of MDS is generally considered to result from the accumulation of **genetic** and non-genetic changes within young blood cells that prevent them from maturing and functioning normally. In MDS, the surrounding cells in the marrow that support the function of blood cells may also be abnormal. However, we do not understand very well how these changes develop and why particular individuals develop them. There are, however, a few clear-cut factors that can influence development of MDS. In some patients who have received **chemotherapy** or **radiation therapy** for a prior cancer, the bone marrow is damaged by the treatment itself, resulting in MDS.

Genetic

occurring within the genes.

Chemotherapy

treatment involving the use of chemical agents, usually for cancer.

Radiation therapy

treatment, usually for cancer, involving the use of radioactive substances to kill diseased cells.

Substantial occupational exposure to toxins such as benzene can increase the risk of developing MDS and AML. MDS related to chemotherapy, radiation therapy, or benzene exposure is frequently associated with an abnormal bone marrow **chromosome analysis** (see Question 19), and the **prognosis** in these cases is poor.

7. Is MDS a cancer?

The issues surrounding this question are well-articulated in a paper by Dr. David Steensma of the Mayo Clinic.[3] Most investigators who study MDS consider it a form of blood/marrow cancer that arises from a sick bone marrow. Others who may not specifically call it a cancer still use terms to describe MDS such as **malignant**, **neoplastic**, and **clonal**. All of these terms are used to describe cancer, or are used to indicate the potential of MDS to evolve to the cancer AML.

Clonal conditions start when a cell mutates and becomes an abnormal cell that "clones" itself, or in other words, one that reproduces to create more abnormal cells. The changes in these cells sometimes occur in the chromosomes and can be identified by chromosome analyses (see Question 19). In the case of MDS, these abnormal cells are young blood cells in the bone marrow that do not mature normally, and they subsequently interfere with the ability of the marrow to produce normal red blood cells, white blood cells, and platelets. Over time, the abnormal cells may come to represent a large proportion of the marrow cell population, ultimately turning into AML.

Chromosome analysis

an examination of chromosomes in a cell to look for abnormalities, structural changes, or extra or missing chromosomes.

Prognosis

projected course of a disease in a particular patient based upon the factors in the individual's health history and in the nature of the disease itself.

Malignant

referring to cancerous cells that invade local tissue or tissue(s) outside the area of origin.

Neoplastic

cancerous or having the potential to develop into cancer.

Clonal

referring to an abnormal cell that reproduces itself.

---

[3]Steensma DP. Are myelodysplastic syndromes "cancer"? Unexpected adverse consequences of linguistic ambiguity. *Leuk Res* 2006; 30:1227–1233.

A useful comparison to understand the cancerous potential of MDS is what can occur with colon polyps. Colon polyps are a collection of abnormal cells that in many instances are found to be **benign** when viewed under the microscope—that is, they are not capable of spreading or invading other parts of the body. However, some polyps may consist of cells that appear more aggressive (pre-malignant or pre-cancerous polyps), or the cells may exhibit outright features of cancer, such as invasion of the wall of the colon. Thus, colon polyps can range across a spectrum from benign, non-cancerous growths, to potentially cancerous, to malignant. Extending this analogy to MDS, dysplastic cells can represent a spectrum from mild to more advanced forms of bone marrow failure, which have the potential to develop into AML. However, because only 30%–40% of MDS patients actually progress to AML, it is no longer considered accurate to call MDS "preleukemia," as it has been called in the past, because it isn't certain that a given patient, particularly one with low-risk disease, will develop leukemia.

The World Health Organization (WHO) (which classifies cancers of the blood/marrow and lymphatic system), the U.S. Food and Drug Administration (FDA), National Cancer Institute, and agencies that provide grants to researchers to study MDS all consider MDS a disease that has biological characteristics of a cancer. However, you should know that some underwriters of health insurance still do not consider MDS a cancer, which has troublesome implications for MDS patients who seek health coverage for treatment of MDS. Multiple reasons exist for the lagging recognition of MDS as a cancer by selected insurance carriers. Regardless, if

Benign

noncancerous.

Only 30%–40% of MDS patients actually progress to leukemia.

you have a diagnosis of MDS, consider reviewing your insurance coverage and discussing the financial situation with your insurance agent, human resources department (if insured through an employer), or a financial management specialist.

Although use of the term "cancer" is laden with heavy negative emotional overtones for patients, including immediate thoughts of death, it is important to obtain specific information regarding *your* prognosis, which is best gauged by the **International Prognostic Scoring System** (**IPSS**; see Question 18). Patients can live with MDS for years, and in lower-risk patients, no treatment may be needed. In fact, because of the older age of most MDS patients, individuals may die *with* MDS, not *from* MDS, because of co-existing medical problems, or simply from old age.

Christine's comments:

When I was first diagnosed with MDS I had never heard of the disease, so I looked it up on the Internet. I was very frightened by the words "smoldering leukemia." My father was a pediatric hematologist and I knew that leukemia was a terminal illness. Then I got printed information from the MDS Foundation. In this information, the word "cancer" was used. This scared me more. The way I dealt with the fear was with explanation and facts: My hematologist suggested that I make an appointment to discuss the diagnosis. She explained what MDS was. She also said that the likelihood of my MDS becoming leukemia was low in view of my FAB classification (RARS). She said that there would be signs ahead of time if my condition was getting worse. Having information helped diminish my fears. Later, I joined an MDS support group. Being able to speak with other people

The Basics

International Prognostic Scoring System (IPSS)
a method of estimating risk of transformation to AML and overall survival for MDS patients.

Patients can live with MDS for years.

with MDS is helpful. So now, I try to concentrate on the present instead of worrying about the future.

8. What is acute myelogenous leukemia (AML)? Can MDS evolve into AML?

Acute myelogenous leukemia (AML) is a cancer of the white blood cells in which immature cells called blasts (see Questions 9 and 11) reproduce rapidly in the bone marrow and do not mature into normal cells. At the same time, the rapid production of cancerous white cells suppresses production of both red cells and platelets in the marrow, leaving the patient anemic and susceptible to bleeding (as well as to infection, as the abnormal white cells cannot fight infection or disease). AML is therefore an extremely serious illness.

MDS progresses to AML in approximately 30%–40% of patients. The time to developing AML varies; some patients move slowly toward AML, some rapidly, and some don't develop AML at all. Certain factors enable physicians to estimate the risk of developing AML, and these factors can be plugged into a scoring system called the International Prognostic Scoring System (IPSS; see Question 18) to help them gauge how long any one person (on average) might have before the transformation from MDS to AML. The development of AML is usually heralded by declining blood cell counts, which may happen gradually or more suddenly. A bone marrow that shows 20% or greater leukemia cells (blasts) formally establishes the diagnosis of AML by the WHO classification. The 20% cut-off is an arbitrary threshold that **hematologists** use to distinguish high-risk MDS from AML.

Acute myelogenous leukemia

a cancer affecting blood cells in which blasts reproduce rapidly but do not mature into normal white blood cells. This often occurs in conjunction with decreased red blood cells and platelets.

Hematologist

a physician who studies blood diseases and disorders.

9. What blood cells does a normal bone marrow make? How is the bone marrow affected in MDS?

In adults, the bone marrow is the site of production of white blood cells, red blood cells, and platelets. **Hematopoietic stem cells**, which are the parent cells of the marrow, constitute a very small percentage of all cells within the marrow, but they are capable of duplicating themselves (self-renewal), and they give rise to all blood cell types. Under the microscope, the youngest recognizable white blood cell in the bone marrow is termed a **blast** (see Question 11).

Blasts give rise to white blood cells of either the **myeloid** type or **lymphoid** type. The most mature type of myeloid white blood cell is named a **neutrophil**. Developing red blood cells within the bone marrow are termed **erythroid precursors**, and developing platelets within the marrow are referred to as **megakaryocytes**.

MDS is frequently characterized by poor maturation of cells within the bone marrow. When cells do not mature properly in the bone marrow, it translates into an inability of the bone marrow to produce sufficient numbers of fully developed, normal white blood cells, red blood cells, or platelets. One perplexing finding in MDS is the fact that some patients have low blood counts even though the bone marrow is packed with cells. This is related to a phenomenon of premature cell death or **apoptosis**. Despite normal or increased numbers of marrow cells being produced, the cells die prematurely and never have the opportunity to leave the marrow and circulate into the blood. Clinically,

The Basics

Hematopoietic stem cells

rare parent cells in the bone marrow that give rise to all blood cells.

Blast

an immature white blood cell.

Myeloid

any white blood cell that is not a lymphocyte (e.g., neutrophils, eosinophils).

Lymphoid

referring to the lymphatic system or lymphocytes—white blood cells that are a part of the lymphatic system and circulate in the blood.

Neutrophil

a mature myeloid white blood cell that is usually a first responder to bacterial or fungal infection.

Erythroid precursors

young, developing red blood cells found in the bone marrow.

Megakaryocytes

a developing cell in the bone marrow that gives rise to platelets in the blood.

Apoptosis

cell death.

Leukopenia

a low total white blood cell count.

Neutropenia

a low neutrophil count.

Thrombocytopenia

a low platelet count.

Cytopenia(s)

a low count of one or more blood cell types.

Leukocyte

any type of white blood cell.

this presents itself as a low total white blood cell count (**leukopenia**), a low neutrophil count (**neutropenia**), a low red blood cell count (anemia), a low platelet count (**thrombocytopenia**), or a combination of these low blood counts (**cytopenias**).

10. What are the functions of white blood cells, red blood cells, and platelets?

The bone marrow carries out several functions, including the production of the three major types of blood cells: white blood cells (also known as **leukocytes**), red blood cells, and platelets (Table 1). Although several different types of white blood cells are produced by the

TABLE 1   Summary of Blood Cells

Name	Light Micrograph	Description	Concentration (Number of Cells/mm³)	Life Span	Function
Red blood cells (RBCs)		Biconcave disk; no nucleus	4–6 million	120 days	Transports oxygen and carbon dioxide
White blood cells Neutrophil		Approximately twice the size of RBCs; multi-lobed nucleus; clear-staining cytoplasm	3000 to 7000	6 hours to a few days	Phagocytizes bacteria
Eosinophil		Approximately same size as neutrophil; large pink-staining granules; bilobed nucleus	100 to 400	8–12 days	Phagocytizes antigen-antibody complex; attacks parasites
Basophil		Slightly smaller than neutrophil; contains large, purple cytoplasmic granules; bilobed nucleus	20 to 50	Few hours to a few days	Releases histamine during inflammation
Monocyte		Larger than neutrophil; cytoplasm grayish-blue; no cytoplasmic granules; U- or kidney-shaped nucleus	100 to 700	Lasts many months	Phagocytizes bacteria, dead cells, and cellular debris
Lymphocyte		Slightly smaller than neutrophil; large, relatively round nucleus that fills the cell	1500 to 3000	Can persist many years	Involved in immune protection, either attacking cells directly or producing antibodies
Platelets		Fragments of megakaryocytes; appear as small dark-staining granules	250,000	5–10 days	Play several key roles in blood clotting

bone marrow, one type, called the neutrophil, is particularly important in fighting bacterial and fungal infections. Red blood cells contain the molecule **hemoglobin**, which transports oxygen to different organs in the body, such as the heart and lungs. Oxygen is critical to the optimal functioning of the body's organs, so anything that affects the number of red blood cells in the circulation also affects the availability of oxygen and, consequently, alters the body's ability to function normally. Platelets are small cells that serve as one arm of the body's clotting system. These cells travel to sites of injury and assist in wound healing to reduce bleeding or bruising. All three types of cells circulate in the blood and can be counted by a routine laboratory test called the **complete blood count (CBC)**. The white blood cell count differential specifically counts the different types of white blood cells. The differential can be performed by a machine in the laboratory (referred to as 'auto differential'), and/or by a technician who looks at the cells under a microscope (referred to as 'manual differential').

Hemoglobin

a molecule in red blood cells that is of key importance in transporting oxygen.

Complete blood count (CBC)

a laboratory test that counts the total quantity of blood cells in a blood sample.

The Basics

11. What is meant by the terms "blast" and "leukemia cell"?

In discussions with your hematologist about MDS, the term *blast* will undoubtedly be used. A blast is a very young, immature white blood cell that divides to give rise to more mature cells (Figure 3). Normal blasts are

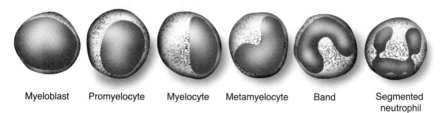

Myeloblast   Promyelocyte   Myelocyte   Metamyelocyte   Band   Segmented neutrophil

Figure 3 The stages of myeloid white blood cell maturation

different from the abnormal blasts that give rise to **leukemia**. Hematologists sometimes refer to the abnormal blasts as *leukemia cells*.

Leukemia

a cancer of the white blood cells.

In normal bone marrow, there is a larger number of mature white blood cells (neutrophils) compared to immature white blood cells, such as blasts; the total quantity of blasts in normal marrow is less than 5%. In MDS, one of the basic abnormalities in the bone marrow is poor maturation of blood cells. Therefore, fewer mature white blood cells may be observed in MDS marrows, and the percentage of immature cells, including abnormal blasts, may increase over time. Additional changes may occur that allow the blasts to multiply, increasing their own numbers instead of producing more mature white blood cells.

The percentage of blasts in the bone marrow is one factor that distinguishes lower-risk versus higher-risk MDS. This is determined by counting the number of blasts present in a group of 100 or 200 white blood cells drawn from a sample of bone marrow.

Lower-risk MDS is generally defined as less than 10% marrow blasts, and higher-risk MDS is defined as 10%–20% marrow blasts. Blasts may also travel from the bone marrow to blood. Therefore, the number of blasts in the blood, if present, may also give an indication as to the severity of MDS. Acute myelogenous leukemia may evolve from MDS, and is defined as the presence of 20% or more marrow blasts in a marrow or blood sample by the World Health Organization (WHO) Classification (see Question 16). Other factors are also considered to determine the severity of each MDS case. These factors include the type and number of chromosome abnormalities found in a bone marrow analysis, and the number of blood cell lines (red blood cells, white blood cells, or platelets) that are decreased. When a blood count is decreased, it is referred to as a cytopenia.

The Basics

PART TWO

Diagnosis, Classification, and Prognosis

Is MDS one disease or a syndrome of similarly related diseases?

How is MDS diagnosed?

What is involved in a bone marrow biopsy? What information does the biopsy provide?

More ...

12. Is MDS one disease or a syndrome of similarly related diseases?

Syndrome

a collection of phenomena seen in association.

Pathologic

indicative of disease or abnormality.

MDS is a syndrome of similarly related diseases of bone marrow failure.

Autoimmune

an immune response against the body's own tissues.

MDS is best classified as a **syndrome** of similarly related diseases of bone marrow failure in which the common clinical feature is low blood counts (especially anemia) and the common **pathologic** feature is dysplasia of one or more blood cell types. Another feature of these similarly related diseases is the potential for changing over time to acute myelogenous leukemia. Despite these shared features, subtypes of MDS may be clinically and biologically different in several respects. Patients may have different clinical presentations of their illness (that is, lower- versus higher-risk MDS, slow versus rapid pace of worsening blood counts, and so on), different factors that may have contributed to the development of marrow failure (for example, environmental, or **autoimmune** attack on the bone marrow as opposed to exposure to prior chemotherapy or radiation), and variable prognoses with regard to overall survival and the risk of developing AML.

Two classification systems—the French-American-British (FAB) and WHO classification systems—have attempted to better define the different subtypes (or syndromes) of MDS, with the goal of providing hematologists and pathologists better specificity in diagnosing and treating these diseases (see Questions 15 and 16).

13. How is MDS diagnosed?

A diagnosis of MDS is based on the finding of one or more low blood counts in conjunction with the finding dysplasia in one or more types of blood cells (usually at least the red blood cells). Dysplasia can also be observed in a sample of the patient's circulating blood cells. Similar to a patient's bone marrow, the patient's blood is smeared on a glass slide and reviewed under a microscope. Because dysplasia can be a consequence of certain drugs, infections, toxins, and alcohol, it is imperative that these factors be eliminated as a cause of dysplasia before labeling a case as MDS.

14. What is involved in a bone marrow biopsy? What information does the biopsy provide?

Although a diagnosis of MDS can be suggested by review of a patient's clinical history, laboratory studies, and review of a slide of the peripheral blood, a bone marrow biopsy is often required to confirm the diagnosis.

As with any medical procedure, a patient's **informed consent** is first obtained by the physician performing the procedure. The **procedurist** will review the informed consent with the patient, describe why the procedure is being done, and outline its potential risks. Patient allergies to medications should also be reviewed at this time. In the case of a bone marrow biopsy, infection and bleeding at the biopsy site are the most common complications, although they are still quite uncommon. If sedatives or narcotics are used before the procedure, it is required that the informed consent be reviewed and signed before these medications are given.

The bone marrow biopsy is an **outpatient** procedure that is typically performed in an exam room in clinic.

A bone marrow biopsy is often required to confirm an MDS diagnosis.

Informed consent

agreement by a patient to a medical procedure after having been carefully informed by the procedurist or hospital of what the purpose, risks, benefits, and nature of the procedure will be.

Procedurist/ Proceduralist

a person who performs a medical procedure and is responsible for describing the procedure to the patient and obtaining informed consent.

Outpatient

not requiring admission into a hospital or other healthcare facility.

Diagnosis, Classification, and Prognosis

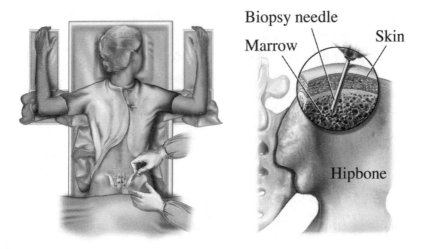

Figure 4 The prone position during a bone marrow biopsy. Illustration copyright 2003 Nucleus Communications, Inc. All rights reserved. http://www.nucleusinc.com.

The patient lies on the exam table either on his or her abdomen (the prone position, Figure 4), or on his or her side. The hip bone on either the patient's right or left back side is the most common site for performing a bone marrow biopsy. The site is approximately 3 fingerbreadths above, and 3 fingerbreadths to the right (or to the left) of the midline of the buttocks. The area of entry on the skin is first cleansed with an antiseptic solution such as with iodine or alcohol swabs. A local anesthetic such as lidocaine is used to numb the skin, the tissue underlying the skin, and the surface of the bone. A small incision is made with a scalpel in the skin for easier entry by the biopsy needles. The first needle, called an **Illinois needle**, is designed for collection of fluid marrow samples. This needle is used to penetrate the surface of the bone (**cortex**) into the marrow space. An anticoagulated syringe is connected to the needle, and the syringe plunger is pulled back to collect the fluid marrow. This fluid is referred to as the **bone marrow aspirate**. Usually 5–10 cc is collected. For clinical trials, additional marrow aspirate may be

Illinois needle

a needle with a syringe fitting for collecting fluid bone marrow.

Cortex

surface of the bone.

Bone marrow aspirate

fluid bone marrow collected during a bone marrow biopsy.

required. One or more insertions of the Illinois needle may be required to collect adequate aspirate. The Illinois needle is removed and a second type of needle, named a **Jamshidi needle**, is used to enter the bone. A middle portion of the Jamshidi needle is removed, and the needle is passed further into the marrow to create a core of solid marrow material (referred to as the **core biopsy**), which moves up the hollow cylinder of the Jamshidi needle. An adequate marrow core biopsy is 1–2 cm in length. To complete the bone marrow biopsy, the procedurist will remove the Jamshidi needle, apply pressure to the biopsy site to minimize bleeding, clean the entry site, and apply clean gauze and/or a bandage.

Dull, achy discomfort related to entry of either type of needle into the skin/tissue and bone marrow is usually felt during the bone marrow biopsy itself. Similar discomfort may also occur with the withdrawal of bone marrow aspirate into the syringe. Sharp pain should be avoidable with the use of the local anesthetic. Discomfort can sometimes last for a few days after the biopsy and should be managed with **acetaminophen**. Generally, aspirin or **non-steroidal anti-inflammatory drugs (NSAIDs)** (ibuprofen or naproxen, for example) should be avoided since these medications can block the function of platelets causing increased bleeding— which is particularly relevant to MDS patients who may have low platelet counts.

The following information from the bone marrow biopsy will be evaluated by a **pathologist**:

Aspirate: The pathologist looks for signs that the red blood cells, white blood cells, and megakaryocytes (platelet precursor cells) are decreased or increased in

Jamshidi needle

a cylindrical needle with a cutting tip designed for collecting core biopsies.

Core biopsy

collection of solid bone marrow material by boring a cylindrical needle into the marrow for a sample.

Acetaminophen

a common pain medication used to treat pain. It is sold over the counter (Tylenol® and other brands) or as a prescription in combination with a narcotic for severe pain.

Non-steroidal anti-inflammatory drugs (NSAIDs)

drugs such as ibuprofen or naproxen used to treat pain, but that should be avoided in patients with MDS with thrombocytopenia because they inhibit platelets.

Pathologist

a physician who examines blood, bone marrow, or other tissue samples to look for signs of disease or dysfunction in the cells.

number. He or she also determines whether the appearance of the cells is abnormal, e.g. there is evidence of dysplasia in the red blood cells or other cell lines. The pathologist also will note whether the blast count is increased, whether stores of iron in the marrow are decreased, normal, or increased, and whether there is evidence of increased **ringed sideroblasts** in the marrow to justify a diagnosis of a subtype of MDS called **refractory anemia with ringed sideroblasts (RARS)** (see Question 15).

Chromosome analysis: A sample of marrow aspirate is sent to the laboratory for chromosome analysis (see Question 19). It usually takes 1–2 weeks for the results to return. Another type of chromosome analysis, referred to as **fluorescent in-situ hybridization (FISH),** can be performed on the marrow aspirate (or peripheral blood). This technique uses color probes directed at specific chromosome segments or specific genes to determine whether they are rearranged, missing, or if additional copies are present.

Flow (immunophenotyping): This technique, performed on the aspirate, sorts individual cells through a column in single file so that specific proteins on the surface of the cells can be identified by lasers and a cocktail of different antibodies directed against the proteins. Because immature cells such as blasts have specific surface markers, flow can be useful as an approach for identifying the percentage of marrow blasts in the marrow.

Core biopsy: The cellularity (composition of cells) of the bone marrow is evaluated. The pathologist can determine whether there are any abnormal cells that

Ringed sideroblasts

red blood cells in the bone marrow that contain characteristic ring-shaped iron deposits.

Refractory anemia with ringed sideroblasts (RARS)

an MDS subtype characterized by the presence of ringed sideroblasts in the bone marrow.

Fluorescent in-situ hybridization (FISH)

a type of chromosome analysis that can determine the presence of abnormal genes or chromosome segments.

have invaded the bone marrow from other sites due to other diseases, including solid tumors such as breast cancer, lymphoma, prostate cancer, and so on. Special stains can be performed on the core biopsy to quantify the percentage of blasts or other populations of cells. Such stains are particularly helpful if the blast count is not available on an aspirate because fluid marrow could not be obtained (the patient has a 'dry tap'). MDS is sometimes associated with scarring of the bone marrow, termed **fibrosis**. The severity of fibrosis can be determined on a core biopsy by using a reticulin and trichrome (collagen) stain.

Fibrosis

scarring of the bone marrow.

15. What is the French–American–British (FAB) Classification of MDS?

Until the 1980s, doctors and researchers used different names to describe what we now commonly recognize as MDS. In addition, there was no agreed-upon method to classify the different subtypes of the disease. In 1982, international investigators published a classification of MDS based on how blood and marrow cells appear under the microscope.[4] This **morphology**-based system for classifying MDS, termed the **French-American-British (FAB) classification**, consists of 5 subtypes of the disease: refractory anemia (RA), refractory anemia with ringed sideroblasts (RARS), refractory anemia with excess blasts (RAEB), refractory anemia with excess blasts in transformation (RAEB-T), and chronic myelomonocytic leukemia (CMML), which is not the same disease as AML but can progress to AML.

Morphology

shape or appearance.

French-American-British classification

a morphology-based MDS classification system published in 1982 by international investigators.

---

[4]Bennett JM, Catovsky D, Daniel MT. Proposals for the classification of the myelodysplastic syndromes. *Br J Haematol* 1982; 51:189–199.

TABLE 2   French–American–British (FAB) Classification of MDS

FAB Subtype	Marrow Blasts	Peripheral Blood Blasts	Comments
Refractory Anemia (RA)	<5%	<1%	<15% ringed sideroblasts
Refractory Anemia with Ringed Sideroblasts (RARS)	<5%	<1%	>15% ringed sideroblasts
Refractory Anemia with Excess Blasts (RAEB)	5%–19%	<5%	
Chronic Myelomonocytic Leukemia (CMML)	0%–19%	<5%	Monocyte count >1000/mm^3 in the peripheral blood
Refractory Anemia with Excess Blasts in Transformation (RAEB-T)	20%–29%	>5%	

Source: Bennett JM, Catovsky D, Daniel MT, et al. Proposals for the classification of the myelo-dysplastic syndromes. *Br J Haematol* 1982; 51:189–199.

As Table 2 shows, a primary factor that distinguishes the various MDS subtypes in the FAB classification is the percentage of bone marrow blasts. Both RA and RARS exhibit less than 5% blasts in the bone marrow. However, RARS is distinguished from RA by the abnormal accumulation of iron in a ring pattern around the nucleus of at least 15% of developing red blood cells in the marrow. These cells, called ringed sideroblasts, can be observed in the bone marrow fluid (aspirate) using a special iron stain. Increasing numbers of blasts within the bone marrow herald more advanced disease. For example, RAEB is defined as 5%–19% marrow blasts, and RAEB–T is defined as 20%–29% blasts in the marrow. In the FAB classification, AML is defined as the presence of 30% or higher marrow blasts.

CMML is a fifth subtype of MDS. It is characterized by an increase in the blood of a particular type of white blood cell called a **monocyte**. A monocyte count of at least 1,000/mm^3 of blood on a complete blood count defines CMML. In addition, the marrow blast count may range from 0% up to 19%. Despite the number of peripheral blood monocytes being increased, CMML may occur with a low, normal, or elevated white blood cell count. CMML has been arbitrarily divided into two subtypes: non-proliferative (dysplastic-type) CMML (white blood cell count ≤12,000/mm^3, recognized by FAB) and proliferative CMML (white blood cell >12,000/mm^3). In addition to the elevated white blood cell count, proliferative-type CMML may be accompanied by other features, including an enlarged liver and spleen.

Monocyte
a white blood cell that is responsible for consuming foreign substances in the body.

The FAB classification can be used to estimate the prognosis of patients with MDS, including a patient's potential for long-term survival and risk of developing AML. In this regard, RA and RARS are considered lower-risk MDS, compared to RAEB-T, which is characterized by poor survival and a high risk of transformation to AML. Depending on the percentage of marrow blasts, RAEB and CMML generally share an intermediate prognosis, but may be relatively better or worse depending on other factors.

16. What is the World Health Organization (WHO) Classification of MDS?

In 2001, the WHO published a new classification of MDS (Table 3) with the goal of providing greater specificity in the pathologic description of MDS and better

TABLE 3   FAB vs. WHO Classification of MDS

FAB	WHO
Refractory anemia (RA)	Refractory anemia with unilineage dysplasia Refractory cytopenia with multilineage dysplasia (RCMD)
—	5q– syndrome
Refractory anemia with ringed sideroblasts (RARS)	RARS with unilineage dysplasia RCMD with ringed sideroblasts
Refractory anemia with excess blasts (RAEB)	RAEB-I (5%–9% BM blasts) RAEB-II (10%–19% BM blasts)
Refractory anemia with excess blasts in transformation (RAEB-T)	Acute myelogenous leukemia (AML)
Chronic myelomonocytic leukemia (CMML)*	Myelodysplastic/myeloproliferative (MDS/MPD) disorder CMML-I (5%–9% BM blasts) CMML-II (10%–19% BM blasts)
—	MDS unclassified

*MDS if WBC count ≤12,000/mm³; MPD if WBC count >12,000/mm³

BM = bone marrow

estimation of prognosis for MDS patients.[5] Compared to the FAB classification, several changes are noted:

1. RAEB-T is eliminated as a subtype, with the new threshold for AML being a blast proportion of 20% or more blasts rather than 30% or more blasts.

2. RA and RARS are each divided into two subtypes, one reflecting the presence of dysplasia in only the red blood cells (**unilineage dysplasia**), and one reflecting dysplasia in more than one cell line (**multilineage dysplasia**).

3. Both RAEB and CMML are subdivided into two subgroups, which partition the percentage of mar-

Unilineage dysplasia

abnormalities of cell shape found in only one cell line, usually red blood cells.

Multilineage dysplasia

abnormalities of cell shape found in more than one cell line.

[5]Brunning RD, Bennett JM, Flandrin G, et al. Myelodysplastic syndromes. In: Jaffe ES, Harris NL, Stein H, Vardiman JW, editors. *World Health Organization classification of tumours. Pathology and genetics. Tumours of hematopoietic and lymphoid tissues, vol. 1.* Lyon, IARC Press; 2001. pp. 62–73.

row blasts into 5%–9% (RAEB-I, CMML-I) and 10%–19% marrow blasts (RAEB-II, CMML-II).

4. **5q– syndrome** is added as a distinct MDS subtype.
5. The category "MDS unclassified" is added for patients with MDS whose disease features don't fit within one of these categories.

5q– syndrome
a subtype of MDS in which patients exhibit a specific chromosome abnormality characterized by loss of a portion of chromosome 5.

The WHO decided to make these changes for the following reasons. First, RAEB-T was eliminated as an MDS disease subtype in the WHO classification because review of the historical prognosis of most of these patients was felt to closely parallel AML patients. However, a minority of patients with RAEB-T will have a considerably more slow-moving course than patients with newly diagnosed AML. Second, a review of the bone marrows and clinical course of MDS patients by hematologists and pathologists found that the number of cell lines exhibiting dysplasia has an impact on prognosis. RA and RARS patients with marrow dysplasia of only the red blood cell line (unilineage dysplasia) have a better prognosis than patients who exhibit dysplasia of more than one cell line (multilineage dysplasia). Third, in the FAB system, CMML and RAEB are defined by a broad range of marrow blasts (0%–19% and 5%–19% blasts, respectively). However, given the importance of the percentage of marrow blasts on prognosis, it is easy to comprehend that an MDS patient with 6% marrow blasts will have a better prognosis than a patient with 16% blasts, with everything else being equal. Therefore, CMML and RAEB are subdivided into Roman numerals I (5%–9% marrow blasts) and II (10%–19% marrow blasts) to call attention to the relatively lower (subtype I) and higher (subtype II) prognostic risk associated with each range of blasts. Finally, the WHO classification added 5q– syndrome, a subtype of MDS in which patients exhibit a specific chromosome abnormality characterized by deletion (loss) of a portion of chromosome 5 and a marrow blast percentage of less than 5%.

Several features are often shared by patients with 5q– syndrome, although some variability exists in the clinical course and presentation. These features are:

1. Relatively good prognosis with long survival and a lower chance of developing acute myelogenous leukemia;
2. Chronic anemia requiring red blood cell transfusions;
3. A slightly higher frequency among women;
4. Elevated platelet count; and
5. Distinct pathologic features on bone marrow specimens, especially involving the platelet precursor cells, megakaryocytes.

After the WHO classification was developed, it was found that the drug lenalidomide is very effective for patients with the 5q– subtype of MDS.

17. Are certain types of MDS not addressed by the FAB and WHO classifications?

Secondary MDS

MDS that develops as a result of prior treatment with chemotherapy or radiation therapy for cancer.

Alkylators

a class of chemotherapy drugs that can sometimes lead to development of MDS or AML.

Three variations of MDS are not formally recognized by the FAB and WHO classifications. **Secondary MDS** refers to MDS that develops as result of prior chemotherapy or radiation treatment (or a combination of the two) for a prior cancer. These therapies can damage the marrow and lead to MDS (or AML). If secondary MDS/AML develops, it typically develops at least 5–10 years after treatment with a class of chemotherapy drugs called **alkylators**. Examples of alkylators include chlorambucil and melphalan. Another class of drugs called **topoisomerase II inhibitors** (for example, etoposide, or VP-16) can lead to MDS/AML in 2–3 years after therapy. Secondary MDS occurs in a minority of patients treated with these drugs, but higher cumulative doses can increase the chances of its development. Patients with secondary MDS generally have a worse prognosis compared to MDS patients who have no prior exposure to chemotherapy or radiation ("de novo MDS"). Also, the IPSS scoring system was developed by analyzing patients only with de novo MDS, and did not include patients with secondary MDS.

Another variant of MDS not included in the FAB or WHO classifications is MDS with fibrosis. Fibrosis refers to the accumulation of either the substance **reticulin** or **collagen** in the bone marrow. Their presence within the marrow can be shown by special stains that pathologists use. The finding of collagen within the bone marrow is a sign of severe fibrosis. Fibrosis is akin to scarring of the bone marrow; it is a reaction to abnormal growth factors produced by cells in the MDS-afflicted marrow. The scarring of marrow replaces the blood cell forming components of the marrow, further contributing to low blood counts. Some literature indicates that MDS with fibrosis is associated with a worse prognosis than MDS not associated with fibrosis. MDS with fibrosis can mimic other diseases of the blood, and in particular, needs to be distinguished from another bone marrow disorder named **primary myelofibrosis**.

With increasing age, the proportion of blood-forming cells in the marrow decreases, and an increasing proportion of the marrow is represented by fat cells. For example, in a 20-year-old individual, normal bone marrow **cellularity** would be 80% blood cells and 20% fat. In an 80-year-old person, normal bone marrow cellularity

Topoisomerase II inhibitors
a class of chemotherapy drugs that can sometimes lead to development of MDS or AML.

Reticulin
a type of structural fiber that crosslinks to form a fine meshwork, which acts as a supporting mesh in soft tissues such as liver, bone marrow, and the tissues and organs of the lymphatic system.

Collagen
the principal protein within connective tissues. Its presence in the bone marrow is a marker of advanced fibrosis.

Primary myelofibrosis
a disorder of the bone marrow sometimes confused with MDS with fibrosis.

Cellularity
the overall cellular composition of a tissue, such as bone marrow.

would be 20% with 80% fat. However, in some patients with MDS, the amount of blood-forming cells in the marrow is abnormally low for their age. This is referred to as hypocellular MDS. An example of this would be a 50-year-old patient with a bone marrow cellularity of 10% blood cells and 90% fat—a far lower proportion of blood cells than one would expect based on age. The bone marrow of hypocellular MDS can appear similar to, and be confused with **idiopathic aplastic anemia**, in which marrow blood cells are destroyed by a person's own immune system, resulting in very low blood counts. The presence of dysplasia and chromosome abnormalities, which are generally not observed with aplastic anemia, can help distinguish the two disorders. However, the similar appearance of hypocellular MDS to aplastic anemia, and several shared biologic features, have led to an appreciation that this form of MDS may also result, in part, from autoimmune attack on the bone marrow. This has led to the use of immunosuppressive drugs to treat hypocellular MDS (see Question 67).

Idiopathic

of unknown origin.

Aplastic anemia

a form of anemia caused by autoimmune attack on the marrow cells.

18. What is the International Prognostic Scoring System (IPSS), and how can I determine my prognosis? What is meant by lower-risk MDS versus higher-risk MDS?

The FAB and WHO classification systems are based on morphology; that is, they categorize MDS based on how the bone marrow and blood appear to pathologists when viewed under a microscope. Clinical hematologists and pathologists work together to determine how the appearance of the marrow (percentage of marrow blasts, dysplasia, etc.) correlates with an individual's risk of developing acute myelogenous leukemia and one's overall survival.

However, the morphology-based FAB and WHO classifications have some potential limitations in estimating risk in MDS. For the most part, these systems do not incorporate important information from examining the chromosomes and do not account for the number of low blood counts, details that can further refine the estimation of a patient's prognosis. The International Prognostic Scoring System (IPSS), developed by Dr. Peter Greenberg and colleagues in 1997, uses three variables—percentage of marrow blasts, chromosomal abnormalities, and number of cytopenias—in order to fine-tune estimates of risk for MDS patients (Table 4).[6]

TABLE 4   International Prognostic Scoring System for MDS

Prognostic Variable	Survival and AML Evolution Score Value				
	0	0.5	1.0	1.5	2.0
Marrow blasts (%)	<5	5–10	—	11–20	21–30
Karyotype[a]	Good	Intermediate	Poor		
Cytopenias[b]	0–1	2–3			

Risk Category	Combined Score
Low	0
Intermediate-1	0.5–1.0
Intermediate-2	1.5–2.0
High	≥2.5

[a]Good = normal, -Y, del(5q), del(20q); poor = complex (≥3 abnormalities) or chromosome 7 anomalies; intermediate = other abnormalities.

[b]Neutrophils <1,800/mm^3, platelets <100,000/mm^3, hemoglobin <10g/dL.

Source: This research was originally published in *Blood.* Greenberg P, et al. International scoring system for evaluating prognosis in myelodysplastic syndromes. *Blood.* 1997; 89:2079–2088. © The American Society of Hematology

[6]Greenberg PL, Cox C, LeBeau MM, et al. International scoring system for evaluating prognosis in myelodysplastic syndromes. *Blood* 1997; 89:2079–2088.

Their analysis was based on the clinical outcomes of over 800 MDS patients who had not received prior treatment, and who did not develop MDS due to prior chemotherapy or radiation (that is, secondary MDS). For each variable, a weight-based score is assigned to the particular marrow blast range (<5%, 5%–10%, 11%–20%, >20%), chromosome subgroup (good, intermediate, or poor), and number of cytopenias (0/1 versus 2/3). A total score is generated from the three variables and can be allocated to one of four risk subgroups: low (total score 0), intermediate-1 (total score 0.5–1.0), intermediate-2 (total score 1.5–2.0), and high (total score ≥2.5). Taken together with age, these subgroups permit a very good estimation of overall survival in years and the number of years it takes for 25% of patients in a particular subgroup to develop AML (Table 5).

The bone marrow biopsy will provide information on the percentage of blasts and chromosomes, unless a good bone marrow specimen could not be obtained. The complete blood count will provide information on how many blood counts are decreased (in other words, whether it is just the red blood cells, or additionally

TABLE 5   Survival and Transformation to AML by IPSS Score*

Parameter	Low	Int-1	Int-2	High
Score	0	0.5–1.0	1.5–2.0	≥2.5
Median Survival, years	5.7	3.5	1.2	0.4
Median AML Transformation, years	9.4	3.3	1.1	0.2

*From diagnosis in untreated patients.

Source: This research was originally published in *Blood.* Greenberg P, et al. International scoring system for evaluating prognosis in myelodysplastic syndromes. *Blood.* 1997; 89:2079–2088. © The American Society of Hematology

the neutrophil count and/or platelet count, that exhibit low counts). You should ask your doctor to review your IPSS score and risk group, and the estimation of overall survival and chance of developing AML. It should be remembered that the IPSS provides estimates of one's survival and risk of developing AML; therefore, any individual patient may exhibit worse or better outcomes compared to those predicted by the IPSS.

19. What are chromosomes, and why is chromosome analysis important in determining the prognosis of MDS patients?

Chromosomes are collections of tightly wrapped stretches of **DNA**, the molecular code that determines how our cells develop. Humans have 46 chromosomes in each cell—22 pairs of chromosomes (numbered 1 to 22), with two additional chromosomes that differ in each gender: men have an X and a Y chromosome, while women have two X chromosomes. Chromosomes are not perfectly symmetrical; they have a long arm denoted by the letter "q" and a short arm denoted by the letter "p." Recent information indicates that a single, entire strand of human DNA (referred to as the **genome**) consists of approximately 30,000 **genes**. Therefore, each chromosome contains, on average, hundreds to thousands of genes. Genes encode proteins that form the basic structure and function of cells. In many diseases, including blood disorders such as MDS, chromosome abnormalities may be observed. As described in Question 14, chromosomes can be visualized and counted in dividing cells from a sample of bone marrow fluid (aspirate).

Chromosome

tightly wrapped chains of DNA. Each human cell has 46 chromosomes.

DNA

deoxyribonucleic acid, the molecule that forms the basis of all genetic information in human cells.

Genome

the complete sequence of human DNA.

Genes

collections of DNA molecules that encode proteins that determine the basic structure and function of living cells.

In a standard bone marrow chromosome analysis, the full set of 46 chromosomes from each of 20 different cells is inspected under a microscope. This is a very small portion of the billions of cells in the bone marrow. During this evaluation, it can be determined whether parts of chromosomes are missing (called **deletions**), and whether these missing parts involve the whole chromosome, or just the long arm (q) or short arm (p) of the chromosome. For example, deletion of the long arm of chromosome 5 is referred to as 5q– (5q minus). However, sometimes chromosomal errors don't involve deletions; in some instances, extra copies of chromosomes may be present forming a triple copy or **trisomy**. For example, when three instead of the normal two copies of chromosome 8 are present, this is referred to as trisomy 8.

Deletions

refers to chromosomes that are missing portions of the genetic code present in normal cells.

Trisomy

presence of an extra copy of a particular chromosome.

The prognosis of MDS patients, specifically overall survival and risk of progressing to AML, is partly related to the findings on chromosome analysis. In addition to percentage of marrow blasts and number of cytopenias, the chromosome evaluation is one of the three factors that have a major impact on prognosis, according to the IPSS. In the IPSS classification, chromosomes are divided into three categories depending on their prognostic risk: good, intermediate, and poor. Table 6 lists the types of chromosome findings in each category.

TABLE 6   Prognosis based on chromosome analysis

Prognosis	Chromosome findings
Good	Normal, 5q– only, 20q– only, Y– only
Intermediate	all other chromosome abnormalities
Poor	–7/7q–, complex chromosome findings (3 or more chromosome abnormalities)

The prognostic significance of other types of chromosome abnormalities has been analyzed by other classification systems in the last several years, and their importance is currently being evaluated.

20. What impact does my age and other medical problems have on MDS, and vice versa?

The advanced age of most MDS patients has several implications. However, it is first important to raise important caveats about age in general. A person who is 70 years old with MDS but has no medical issues aside from MDS may be biologically more "youthful" than a 60-year-old individual with MDS and a 30-year history of smoking who has multiple illnesses such as heart and lung disease. Hematologists therefore need to evaluate the biologic *and* chronologic age of a patient when making treatment decisions. Nevertheless, poor health or advanced age may prevent some patients from receiving certain high-intensity treatments such as chemotherapy or bone marrow/stem cell transplantation. Many transplant centers will not perform a myeloablative stem cell transplantation in a patient greater than age 55 to 60 years old because of the high risk of treatment-related death in older individuals, regardless of whether a patient has overall excellent health (see Question 71).

Patient age may also influence an individual's goals of care. For example, an 80-year-old with high-risk MDS and an expectation of rapid transformation to AML and shortened survival may desire improved quality of life as the primary therapeutic outcome rather than longer life. This may be achieved with supportive care measures such as red blood cell transfusions or hematopoietic growth factors (see Part Four: Treatment, Supportive Care, and Side Effects). In contrast, a 55-year-old confronted with higher-risk MDS may choose a high-intensity therapy such as stem cell transplantation (see Part Five: Stem Cell and Bone Marrow Transplantation) with the goal of trying to cure MDS.

Age does have an additional influence on prognosis in patients with lower-risk MDS. Using two age comparisons of ≤60 years versus >60 years and ≤70 versus >70 years, patients with increased age have worse outcomes. However, age differences do not exert additional influence on the IPSS estimates of survival and time to evolution to AML in patients with higher-risk MDS.

The existence of other medical problems can complicate MDS. Patients with heart and lung disease tend to tolerate anemia less well. As a result, it is common practice to use a higher hemoglobin threshold (that is, at least 9–10 g/dL, instead of 8–9 g/dL) to transfuse red blood cells, in order to lessen symptoms of fatigue and shortness of breath. Additional medical illnesses may complicate tolerance of even basic therapies. A patient with heart failure may require red blood cell transfusions to be run very slowly or may need diuretics to prevent or treat fluid overload. Because certain therapies (hypomethylating agents and chemotherapy) are dosed according to one's level of kidney or liver function, modification of the dose or schedule of these drugs may require adjustment before or during the course of treatment.

PART THREE

Symptoms and Treatment Options

How is response evaluated in MDS?

What are the most common presenting symptoms in MDS?

What factors are weighed when evaluating specific treatment options for MDS?

More ...

21. How is response evaluated in MDS?

Evaluation of the blood counts and bone marrow are essential components to assessing response in MDS. For this reason, it is important to have a recent bone marrow evaluation and blood count as a baseline to judge response before commencing any new therapy.

Evaluation of the complete blood count will allow the doctor to determine whether previously abnormal blood counts have improved. Review of bone marrow studies permits the treating doctor and pathologist to ask the following questions after treatment:

1. If the bone marrow blast percentage was increased before treatment, has it now decreased, returned to normal, or increased further?
2. Has the dysplasia persisted or resolved?
3. If ringed sideroblasts were visible, are they still present and in the same numbers?
4. If prior chromosome abnormalities were present, have they persisted, disappeared, or are new chromosome abnormalities present?
5. Additional bone marrow findings that should be commented upon include the adequacy of iron stores (decreased, increased, or the same during the interval treatment), and the degree of marrow fibrosis, if present.

Until recently, studies used different criteria to define hematologic response in MDS. In 2000, the International Working Group (IWG) in MDS published consensus response criteria to define what constitutes a "response" in the red blood cells, neutrophils, and platelets.[7] For example, a minor red blood cell response was defined as a 1–2 g/dL increase in the hemoglobin level, or a 50% decrease in transfusions in patients dependent on red blood cell transfusions. A major red blood cell response was defined as a >2 g/dL hemoglobin increase or transfusion independence. These benefits must last for at least 2 months in order to meet criteria for response. This requirement was added in order to establish a minimum threshold for response, since a response that lasts for 2 weeks, for example, was not felt to be clinically meaningful. The IWG also defined responses for therapies that have the potential for altering the course of MDS, such as improving survival, delaying transformation to AML, and possibly curing MDS. Categories that fall into this response group include 'complete remission,' 'partial remission,' 'stable disease,' 'progressive disease,' and 'relapse.' In addition to alterations of blood counts, changes in the bone marrow blast percentage and dysplasia are used to judge response.

In 2006, the IWG modified the previously published response criteria to make them even more clinically appropriate to MDS patients and the treatments they receive.[8]

---

[7]Cheson BD, Bennett JM, Kantarjian H, et al. Report of an international working group to standardize response criteria for myelodysplastic syndromes. *Blood* 2000; 96:3671–3674.

[8]Cheson BD, Greenberg PL, Bennett JM, et al. Clinical application and proposal for modification of the International Working Group (IWG) response criteria in myelodysplasia. *Blood.* 2006; 108:419–425.

22. What are the most common presenting symptoms in MDS?

Anemia is the most common laboratory finding when MDS is initially diagnosed. Anemia may be mild and found as an incidental laboratory result when a routine complete blood count is obtained for other reasons. However, when anemia is more severe (usually when hemoglobin levels are less than 10 g/dL), it can lead to fatigue, shortness of breath, and difficulty tolerating exercise or routine physical activites that were previously performed routinely (for example, walking up stairs). Patients often note that these are activities that they had at one time performed seamlessly. However, since the anemia usually develops over months, and sometimes years, the body can accommodate to these changes such that patients may not appreciate significant changes in their energy level, even with exercise.

Severe anemia can lead to fatigue, shortness of breath, and difficulty tolerating exercise or routine physical activity.

A lower percentage of MDS patients exhibit a low white blood cell count (leukopenia) or a low neutrophil count (neutropenia) at the time of diagnosis. When the neutrophil count becomes progressively lower, especially under 500/mm^3, patients may develop recurrent infections (especially bacterial), or infections that linger despite antibiotic treatment.

A low platelet count occurs least commonly as an initial sign of MDS. Bleeding or severe bruising is usually a symptom of severe thrombocytopenia (that is, a platelet count less than 20,000/mm^3). The development of worsening thrombocytopenia to this level often indicates that MDS is evolving from a lower-risk to higher-risk state, or AML.

Symptoms and Treatment Options

Meredith's comment:

I began to notice upon walking with friends up three very steep hills, a walk we did three times a week, that I no longer felt energized by the end of the climb. I was overly tired, breathless, and at times even exhausted. But it was a fast-paced walk up a two-block-long slight rise that sent me to the doctor. My heart was beating too rapidly, I felt nauseated and breathless. Blood tests showed anemia and finally a bone marrow extraction confirmed MDS.

Norma's comment:

I had no idea I was sick. I had blood tests every year, but was told women my age were often anemic. I was 55. Thankfully, my orthopedic surgeon saw that my hemoglobin was 7 and immediately started an investigation. After about five different doctors I was diagnosed with MDS. I had the 5q– deletion.

23. Why am I tired?

Fatigue is a common complaint among MDS patients, and may be related to several factors. MDS-related anemia is a common cause of fatigue. The hemoglobin level that produces fatigue in a patient may vary greatly. In addition, co-existing medical problems such as coronary artery disease, heart failure, lung disease, diabetes, or simply older age may contribute to one's subjective sense of fatigue. Although some of the goals of treatment in MDS include improvement of blood counts, prevention of the onset of AML, and improvement of quality of life, an unintended consequence of some therapies can be new or worsening fatigue. Depression, anxiety, and other psychosocial stressors may also contribute to fatigue during the course of one's battle with MDS. Engaging the help of a psychologist or psychiatrist and/or the use of antidepressants or anti-anxiety medications may help these symptoms. Lastly, fatigue can represent a symptom related to other medical conditions, such as lung or heart disease, diabetes, and low thyroid levels (hypothyroidism).

Millie's comment:

I know that I am unable to do the various chores I once did. I used to take a 45-minute walk up a hill and back at a fast pace. Now I go slower. I also gave up my yoga class to avoid crowds and don't overextend myself. I will go back to yoga at a later date, though, because it is so good for me.

24. How severe is my anemia, and how will it affect me?

Anemia refers to a low red blood cell count in the blood. Red blood cells carry oxygen to vital organs, enabling them to function in an optimal fashion. Approximately 80% of patients with MDS will present with anemia at the time of their diagnosis.

Hematocrit

the proportion of the blood volume that is occupied by red blood cells.

Your hematologist will commonly use two terms to describe the red blood cell count: the hemoglobin (Hb), and the **hematocrit (Hct)**. The hemoglobin is a value directly measured from the blood by laboratory instruments, and the hematocrit is calculated from the hemoglobin. The hematocrit is usually three times the value of the hemoglobin. For example, if a patient has a hemoglobin of 10 g/dL, the hematocrit would be approximately 30. Although a normal range of hemoglobin/hematocrit values exists for men and women, and this reference range varies slightly between labs, an average normal value to remember for men is 15, and an average normal value for women is 13–14. These values are expressed as grams/deciliter (g/dL).

When the Hb/Hct falls below normal range, a patient is referred to as anemic. Mild anemia usually refers to anemia slightly below the normal range, for example 10–13 g/dL. Moderate anemia generally refers to Hb values in the range of 8–10 g/dL. Severe anemia generally refers to Hb values below 8 g/dL.

It is important to remember that there are many causes of anemia. Broadly speaking, anemia is either due to:

1. decreased production of red blood cells by the bone marrow,
2. increased destruction of red blood cells circulating in the blood, termed **hemolysis**,
3. blood loss, usually due to menstrual or gastrointestinal bleeding, and
4. **sequestration**, in which red blood cells become trapped by the spleen due to various illnesses.

Causes of gastrointestinal bleeding or excessive menstrual bleeding (resulting in iron deficiency) require work-up by your doctor(s). The anemia of MDS is due to decreased production of red blood cells by the marrow. Therefore, MDS patients are generally referred to as having a **hypoproductive anemia**. The reticulocyte count is a blood test that measures the number of young red blood cells in the blood. In MDS, the reticulocyte count is usually low for the degree of anemia. The MDS marrow is unable to produce enough young red blood cells to compensate for the anemia. MDS-related anemia is entirely different from iron deficiency or other forms of nutritional deficiency. However, it is still possible that more than one cause of

Hemolysis

destruction of red blood cells in the circulation.

Sequestration

trapping of red blood cells in the spleen due to illness.

Hypoproductive anemia

a form of anemia in which lowered production of red blood cells by the bone marrow is the cause of the low red blood cell count.

43

anemia may simultaneously exist in one patient, and may require further diagnostic work-up and treatment by your doctor.

Anemia affects individuals differently, and the Hb level at which patients begin experiencing symptoms may vary widely. However, as the Hb falls toward 10 g/dL, patients may start experiencing fatigue and shortness of breath. These symptoms may be worsened with activity, such as walking up stairs. Patients may complain of decreased exercise tolerance—that is, individuals are unable to perform exercise or their daily physical routine with the same intensity or endurance as they once could with a normal Hb. Patients may wish to take more frequent naps during the day or sleep longer during the night to recuperate their energy. For patients with pre-existing heart disease (coronary artery disease or congestive heart failure) or lung disease (emphysema, chronic obstructive lung disease [COPD]), anemia may worsen pre-existing symptoms of chest pain and shortness of breath. Other symptoms of anemia that patients may describe include lightheadedness, difficulty with memory or clear thinking, and less clear vision.

25. How severe is my low neutrophil count (neutropenia), and how will it affect me?

A primary function of white blood cells is to fight infection. In normal individuals, the total white blood cell count, also referred to as the total leukocyte count, is approximately 4,000–11,000/mm^3, although the normal range may vary slightly between laboratories. There are several different types of white blood cells, which serve different functions within the immune system. One type of white blood cell, named the neutrophil, is important for fighting bacterial infections. MDS patients may develop a low leukocyte count (leukopenia) and neutrophil count (neutropenia). Hematologists often refer to the **absolute neutrophil count**, or **ANC**, to describe the total neutrophil count in the blood.

The lower limit of the normal neutrophil range is approximately 1500/mm^3. An ANC of 1000–1500/mm^3 is considered mild neutropenia; 500–1000/mm^3 is moderate neutropenia, and less than 500/mm^3 is severe neutropenia. The International Prognostic Scoring System (IPSS) defines an ANC less than 1800/mm^3 as neutropenia.

The risk of developing a life-threatening infection increases as the ANC decreases, and the risk is especially high with an ANC below 500/mm^3. A patient with neutropenia who develops a fever should consider it a medical emergency because the body's immune system may not be able to fight infection; what might be a minor illness in a healthy person could, in a neutropenic person, potentially result in death. A patient with neutropenia who develops a fever should immediately contact his or her doctor or go to the hospital for urgent evaluation to obtain blood tests, blood cultures to search for an infection in the blood (bacteremia), a chest x-ray to evaluate for pneumonia, and a urinalysis and urine culture to rule out a urinary tract infection. Antibiotics should be started immediately after the blood and urine specimens have been collected. In most cases, patients will be admitted to the hospital for intravenous antibiotics, and will be hospitalized until the fever/infection and symptoms improve.

Absolute neutrophil count (ANC)
an estimation of the total number of neutrophils in the blood. The ANC is calculated by multiplying the total white blood cell (WBC) count times the percentage of neutrophils.

A patient with neutropenia who develops a fever should immediately contact his or her doctor.

26. How severe is my low platelet count, and how will it affect me?

Platelets are small cells in the blood that are important for clotting blood. The normal platelet count in the blood is 150,000–400,000/mm^3. A low platelet count is referred to as thrombocytopenia.

Similar to anemia and neutropenia, there are varying degrees of thrombocytopenia. Mild thrombocytopenia may be arbitrarily defined as a platelet count of 100,000–150,000/mm^3; moderate thrombocytopenia as 50,000–100,000/mm^3; and severe thrombocytopenia as less than 50,000/mm^3.

Many prescription, over-the-counter, and herbal medications may reduce the platelet count or block platelet function, so you and your doctor should review the medications you take.

As the platelet count falls below 50,000/mm^3, but particularly below 10,000–20,000/mm^3, the risk of bleeding or bruising increases substantially. Bleeding may become evident as nosebleeds, gum bleeding, blood in the urine, or bloody or dark/tarry stools or tiny purple spots under the skin, referred to as petechaie. Bleeding in the brain (a hemorrhagic stroke) is a potentially fatal complication. Skin bruising may occur spontaneously, or be provoked by simple accidents, such as bumping into furniture. Skin bruising may also turn into hematomas, which are raised collections of blood in the skin or soft tissues.

When severe thrombocytopenia develops, you should avoid taking aspirin or NSAIDs (e.g., Advil, Aleve, Motrin, and similar over-the-counter medications). These medicines can block the clotting function of platelets and contribute to increased bleeding. Blood thinners such as warfarin (Coumadin) or anti-platelet drugs such as clopidogrel (Plavix) should also be avoided. Many prescription and over-the-counter medications may also either reduce the platelet count or block their function, so you and your doctor should review the medications you take . Elective surgeries and dental procedures should be approached with caution, or alternatively postponed or cancelled, in patients with severe thrombocytopenia because of the increased risk of bleeding. If such procedures are essential, discuss the use of platelet transfusions before, during, and after the procedure with your hematologist and the surgeon/dentist. In addition to a reduced platelet count, the clotting function of platelets may also be abnormally affected in MDS (**thrombocytopathy**). Therefore, MDS patients may still experience bleeding or bruising even when platelet counts are not as low as one might anticipate for the severity of symptoms.

Thrombocytopathy

a decrease in the ability of platelets to perform the clotting function.

27. What factors are weighed when evaluating specific treatment options for MDS?

Three factors play a primary role in the decision making process about treatment in MDS: IPSS score, **performance status**, and age. Issues related to age are discussed in Question 20.

Performance status

a patient's overall health and ability to function.

Several patient scenarios demonstrate the interplay of these factors. In scenario #1, for a 65-year-old man who falls in the low IPSS subgroup (no increased marrow blasts, only mildly symptomatic anemia [e.g., Hb 9.5 g/dL], and normal chromosomes), the use of red blood cell injections with red blood cell transfusions as needed is a very appropriate treatment plan. In scenario #2, for an otherwise healthy 65-year-old man with intermediate-2 IPSS subgroup (12% marrow blasts, anemia, a low neutrophil count, and normal chromosomes), the use of hypomethylating therapy (such as 5-azacitidine or decitabine) in order to delay the progression to leukemia would be a reasonable management course. In scenario #3, an 85-year-old man with intermediate-2 IPSS subgroup has the same MDS features as the patient in scenario #2, but is functionally very weak (poor performance status), and his kidney and liver function are severely compromised. In this case, the patient may not be able to tolerate the optimal doses of hypomethylating therapy. Although transformation to AML is a near-term possibility, his goals of care may be focused on quality of life. In scenario #4, a 53-year-old woman with MDS has the same intermediate-2 IPSS subgroup. She has good overall health and a sister who is found to be a suitable **HLA-matched donor**. In this case, the presence of advanced MDS, good overall health, and the availability of an HLA-matched sibling make **stem cell transplantation** a reasonable treatment option. Your doctor will weigh your IPSS, age, performance status, and goals of care when balancing the benefits and risks of the care plan being proposed.

HLA-matched donor

an individual whose human leukocyte antigens (HLA) match those of a sick person such that a transplantation of healthy cells from the donor is feasible.

Stem cell transplantation

transplantation of stem cells from another individual into a person with a bone marrow disorder or other disease.

28. What are the broad categories of treatment available in MDS?

Treatment in MDS can be categorized in different ways, but mechanism of action is one useful method to distinguish available therapies. Based on mechanism of action, therapies for MDS can be divided into hematopoietic growth factors, immunomodulatory/anti-angiogenic agents, hypomethylating drugs, anti-immune agents, chemotherapy, bone marrow/stem cell transplantation, iron chelators, and supportive care. Table 7 lists examples of therapies under each category.

TABLE 7   Drugs Used in MDS.

Class of Drug/ Mechanism of Action	Generic Name	Brand Name(s)	Comments
Supportive care			Red blood cell and platelet transfusions, antibiotics
Hematopoietic growth factor	Erythropoietin (EPO)	Procrit Epogen	
	Darbepoetin	Aranesp	
	Granulocyte-Colony Stimulating Factor (G-CSF)	Neupogen	
Immunomodulatory/ anti-angiogenic drug	Lenalidomide	Revlimid	FDA-approved for low/int-1 transfusion-dependent 5q– MDS
Hypomethylating agent	5-azacitidine	Vidaza	FDA-approved for all FAB subtypes of MDS
	Decitabine	Dacogen	FDA-approved for all FAB subtypes of MDS
Immunosuppressive therapy	Horse or rabbit anti-thymocyte globulin (ATG); cyclosporine		
Chemotherapy	Cytarabine, idarubicin, fludarabine, topotecan		
Stem cell/bone marrow transplantation			Donor source: Allogeneic (matched sibling or unrelated donor) vs. autologous vs. cord blood
			Conditioning regimen intensity: myeloablative vs. reduced intensity vs. non-myeloablative
Iron chelator	Deferasirox	Exjade	FDA-approved for the treatment of chronic iron overload due to blood transfusions (includes MDS)
	Deferoxamine	Desferal	

29. When would my doctor recommend "watch and wait" as a management plan?

In the IPSS-designated low-risk subgroup of MDS patients, only very mild decreases in one or more blood counts may be present. This group of patients also has either normal chromosomes or low-risk chromosomal changes on bone marrow analysis, and no increased marrow blasts. As an example, a hemoglobin level of 12 g/dL may be found in a male MDS patient whose normal hemoglobin level should be in the range of 14–16 g/dL. However, this mild decrease in hemoglobin is not expected to cause anemia-related symptoms such as fatigue or shortness of breath. Also, unless the patient is an athlete or well-conditioned, changes in exercise endurance are unlikely to be apparent. Therefore, red blood cell transfusions or red blood cell injections to improve the mild anemia are not medically warranted. A "watch and wait" approach is an appropriate management plan in this case. This involves waiting to begin therapy, but also watching for any concerning changes in the blood counts by obtaining blood tests every several months (or an interval to be decided by the hematologist). If worse blood counts should emerge, a bone marrow biopsy may be necessary to understand the reason for these trends. Sometimes, increased marrow blasts or new chromosome abnormalities may be found, indicative that MDS is progressing to a higher-risk state. Despite having lower-risk disease and no need for treatment, the notion of a "watch and wait" approach can be unsettling to some patients. Not actively engaging in treatment may make patients feel passive and helpless.

PART FOUR

Treatment, Supportive Care, and Side Effects

What is the difference between treatment and supportive care? What are the components of each option?

When do I need a red blood cell transfusion?

What does it mean if I develop antibodies to red blood cells or platelet transfusions?

Is there a role for chemotherapy in the treatment of MDS?

More ...

30. What is the difference between treatment and supportive care? What are the components of each option?

Treatment of MDS is intended to prolong the patient's life and improve quality of life. Obviously, the best way to do this is to cure the disease, but when a disease is incurable—or when the strategies to obtain the cure are more dangerous to the patient than the disease itself, as is sometimes the case in MDS—treatment strategy focuses on controlling the disease's progression and enhancing patients' physical and emotional well-being. Treatment strategies for MDS include the use of potentially curative therapies such as stem cell or bone marrow transplantation, which are discussed in Part Five. When these therapies are considered too risky (that is, more likely to cause the patient's death than the MDS), treatment consists of a combination of drug therapy and supportive care. **Supportive care** refers to therapies that aim to improve the patient's quality of life without specifically treating the MDS. In some patients, the therapies available for treatment cause so many severe side effects that the patients are either unable or unwilling to tolerate them; elderly patients or patients with other existing illnesses, for example, may find that extending their lives by treating MDS simply isn't worth the side effects they would experience. In these situations, it is more appropriate to give supportive care without MDS-specific treatment so that the patient is comfortable.

Supportive care consists of transfusions, antibiotics, and pain medications. For example, red blood cell transfusions may be administered to improve symptoms of fatigue and shortness of breath. Platelet trans-

Supportive care

care intended to improve quality of life without necessarily directly treating the disease.

fusions may be administered to prevent or treat bleeding symptoms. For patients with active infection, antibiotics (either oral or intravenous) are given. Sometimes a doctor may prescribe antibiotics if a patient has a history of recurrent infections and a low neutrophil count—these are termed **prophylactic** antibiotics.

Prophylactic

a medication or treatment intended as a preventative for a likely complication.

Because supportive care is given to patients regardless of whether they receive treatment for MDS, we will discuss supportive care measures first, then describe treatment. Curative treatment through transplantation is discussed in a separate section (Part Five).

SUPPORTIVE CARE

31. When do I need a red blood cell transfusion?

Red blood cell transfusions are indicated for a patient when he or she becomes **symptomatic** from anemia. The level of hemoglobin that elicits symptoms of fatigue and/or shortness of breath varies between individuals, and may partly depend on the patient's age, other illnesses, and the rate of decline of the hemoglobin. For example, an individual who experiences a very slow and gradual decline in the hemoglobin over several months to years may be able to accommodate him- or herself to a low hemoglobin level, whereas an individual whose hemoglobin decreases to the same level in only a few weeks or days might be unable to adjust. Patients with active coronary artery disease, heart failure, or lung disease may develop symptoms related to their anemia at a relatively higher level of hemoglobin compared to other patients who are otherwise healthy and of the same age.

Symptomatic

showing apparent effects of an illness or disorder.

The schedule of red blood cell transfusions will be dictated by the severity of a patient's anemia-related symptoms and the level of hemoglobin in the blood. You may receive transfusions weekly, every two weeks, or every three weeks, depending on your hemoglobin levels and the type of response that is seen. Red blood cell transfusions are associated with improvement in anemia-related symptoms and quality of life. Patients who are on a fixed schedule of red blood cell transfusions commonly report that their anemia-related symptoms return before their next set of transfusions. If you are experiencing fatigue and shortness of breath most of the time between transfusions, either the hemoglobin threshold for administering transfusions should be increased, or the frequency of transfusions should be increased, or both.

32. What is involved in getting a red blood cell transfusion, and what are the risks to me?

If you and your physician decide that you would benefit from transfusions, you will have a blood specimen drawn for blood typing and cross matching. Once your blood type is known, one or more units of blood with the same type are chosen to be tested for cross matching to see if the particular units chosen are compatible with your blood. Depending on the facility where you are receiving the transfusion and whether blood with your type is available, this process can take as little as 2 hours or as long 1 or 2 days.

Transfusion reaction

a reaction in the patient who receives red blood cells or platelets. Transfusion reactions may have different causes.

Cross matching the donor blood with your own blood greatly decreases the chances of your body reacting to the foreign blood in what is called a **transfusion reaction**, which is the principal risk associated with blood transfusions. Transfusion reactions can range from being mild (hives, rash, itching), to moderate (fever, low blood pressure, shortness of breath), and very rarely life-threatening (requiring transfer to the intensive care unit because of compromise of heart or lung function). Many physicians will prescribe medication to be taken about 30 minutes before a blood transfusion. These "pre-medications" are commonly acetaminophen (Tylenol®) and diphenhydramine hydrochloride (Benadryl®), and in some cases, hydrocortisone. These pre-medications can further decrease the chances of a transfusion reaction.

Transfusions are usually given through an **intravenous (IV) needle** placed in the arm. The needle used for transfusions are a little bit bigger than needles used to infuse antibiotics or hydration fluids. Transfusions can also be given through venous access devices such as a PICC line or port. The process usually takes 2 to 2½ hours per unit. Some facilities can give transfusions to outpatients, but some facilities require the patient be admitted to the hospital. Transfusions are not given at home by home-care agencies or hospice care.

Intravenous (IV) needle

a tube inserted into a vein to allow direct injection of medication.

The risk of contracting a disease from transfusions is extremely small.

Many people feel concern about the risk of contracting a disease from transfusions. In fact, this risk is extremely small. The blood you receive during a red blood cell transfusion can come from one of two sources. Most blood will come from that donated by unpaid volunteers. The volunteer donors are screened first by answering questions regarding their medical history. The medical history will include questions about their sexual habits, drug use, and recent travel. If they pass the medical history screening, their blood is taken and tested for blood-borne infections like HIV and hepatitis. Though this process can never guarantee that all blood is 100% free of contagious diseases, the risk is extremely low. HIV and hepatitis C infection is carried in less than one in 2,000,000 units of blood, and hepatitis B occurs in about one in 250,000 transfused units. Like viral infections, bacterial infections are rare but can be life threatening.

The second source for blood is from designated donors. Designated donors are friends or relatives of the patient who have agreed to give blood specifically for use by the patient. There is no proof that this method is safer than using the blood from the volunteer donors. In fact, designated donor blood may carry more risk of carrying viral infections because friends and family members may be less inclined to admit that they have engaged in behaviors such as intravenous drug use or some sexual behaviors that increase their chances of carrying an infection.

Discuss all risks and benefits of blood transfusions with your doctor before deciding whether transfusions are right for you.

Meredith's comment:

The week or so before getting my first transfusion was filled with anxiety about pain, the future, iron overload, everything. But the event itself was, as were all the following transfusions, one of reassurance, calmness, comfort, and even humor. The nurses in the transfusion/ infusion rooms are professionals: reassuring, kind, warm-hearted, sympathetic, and matter-of-fact. I cannot speak highly enough of them, and I have heard the exact same impression from other MDS patients.

33. How frequently will I need platelet transfusions?

Platelet transfusions are given for bleeding symptoms associated with a low platelet count. Platelet transfusions are typically called for when a patient has moderate bleeding from the nose or mouth or gastrointestinal bleeding. In some cases, if the patient has no symptoms but the platelet count is below a certain threshold, a platelet transfusion may be ordered to prevent the possibility of bleeding symptoms. In MDS patients, a platelet count in the range of 10,000–20,000/mm^3 usually indicates very severe disease and might indicate that transformation to AML has occurred.

For the patient with bleeding symptoms, the frequency of platelet transfusions will depend on the frequency of bleeding symptoms and their severity. In patients who have low platelet counts but no active bleeding, the frequency of transfusions may vary from weekly to three times weekly. Transfused platelets have a short lifespan (only 3–5 days), so regular platelet transfusions are needed to keep platelet counts in a safe range. However, because of the concern that the patient might develop resistance after repeated platelet transfusions (see Question 34), some physicians may choose to administer platelet transfusions only when bleeding symptoms develop, and not just for a platelet count below 10,000–20,000/mm^3. The greatest risk from a low platelet count is bleeding in the brain, called a hemorrhagic stroke.

34. What does it mean if I develop antibodies to red blood cells or platelet transfusions?

Some patients develop antibodies to transfused blood products in a process referred to as **alloimmunization**; that is, the immune system recognizes certain components of the transfused blood cells as foreign and reacts by destroying them. As a result, the transfused red blood cells or platelets are quickly destroyed and do not benefit the patient.

Alloimmunization

the development of antibodies against red blood cells or platelets that can occur with repeated red blood cell or platelet transfusions, respectively. This can lead to difficulty finding compatible red blood cell units for transfusion or resistance to platelet transfusions.

When a patient starts requiring more blood products, antibody development is one of the possible causes a physician will explore. Your physician may perform a blood draw one hour after a platelet transfusion to determine whether the platelet transfusion has resulted in an adequate rise in the platelet count. If not, use of 'HLA-matched' platelets may be recommended. Your hematologist/oncologist will submit a sample of your blood to the transfusion services lab for an antibody screen or compatibility test. If the test is positive for antibodies, your transfusion services lab may be able to locate a volunteer donor whose cells do not carry the antigens your body has developed antibodies against. If such a donor is found, they may be called to donate blood products for you. 'HLA-matched' donor platelets, which are platelets very similar to the patient's, may be used in an attempt to overcome the antibodies that have developed; with matched platelets, the body can be fooled into accepting the donor platelets as belonging to the patient. Increasing the dose or number of pre-medications (acetaminophen, diphenhydramine, and hydrocortisone) may also help reduce the chance of a reaction to the transfused blood products.

35. How does the excess iron from red blood cell transfusions affect my body?

MDS patients who suffer from anemia and require regular red blood cell transfusions are at risk for developing **iron overload**. Each unit of red blood cells contains approximately 200–250 mg of iron. Iron loss of 1–2 mg occurs naturally on a daily basis through loss of superficial cells that line the gastrointestinal tract, and through menstruation in premenopausal women. However, the body has no additional mechanism to remove the excess iron from red blood cell transfusions, and signs of iron overload can be observed after 10 to 20 transfusions. Iron overload can damage organs, particularly the heart, liver, and pancreas, and this damage can lead to premature death. For example, progressive iron overload in the heart can result in heart failure and abnormal heart rhythms. Changes in the liver can range from mild liver function abnormalities to cirrhosis and liver failure. Accumulation of iron in the pancreas can lead to diabetes. It can also cause non-life-threatening health problems such as infertility, skin discoloration, and arthritis. All of these problems can be determined through various tests. Blood testing is used to assess liver function. The development of diabetes can also be assessed by blood tests, including measurement of a fasting blood sugar. Heart function can be assessed by various tests, including an electrocardiogram (EKG) and heart ultrasound (echocardiogram).

Iron overload

excessive quantities of iron in the blood, which may lead to organ damage.

36. What medicines are available to remove iron from the body? When is the right time to start using them?

Iron chelator

a medication that removes excess iron from the blood.

Serum ferritin

a blood test which measures the amount of storage iron in the body.

If iron overload becomes a problem for you, your physician will prescribe drugs called **iron chelators** to remove excess iron from the blood. The need for iron chelators usually develops after 20–30 red blood cell transfusions; your doctor will use your **serum ferritin** level to determine whether you're in danger of experiencing iron overload. He or she will watch for serum ferritin levels approaching 2000–2500 ng/mL. At the same time, your doctor will monitor your organ function so that if abnormalities related to iron overload develop before you reach the range of 2000–2500 ng/mL (as sometimes happens), the iron chelators can be employed to prevent serious organ damage before it occurs.

One such drug, deferoxamine (brand name Desferal®), has been available as an iron chelator for over 30 years. Although this medicine can be very effective in reducing iron overload when used to its full extent, it has one major drawback: because of its short half-life in the blood, it must be administered 5–7 days weekly for 8 to 12 hours using a pump that transfers the drug into an injection site under the skin in order to be most effective. This difficult dosing method often causes patients to be unwilling to follow the treatment schedule despite knowing the potential dangerous effects of iron overload.

An alternative treatment for transfusion-related iron overload, deferasirox (brand name Exjade®), is now FDA-approved for use in several diseases associated with this condition. Deferasirox is available as a tablet that is dissolved in water and taken half an hour after food once daily. A standard dose of deferoxamine (40 mg/kg) versus deferasirox 20 mg/kg (tested in patients with B-thalassemia, an unrelated disease with similar symptoms), showed equivalent ability to reduce the serum ferritin and liver iron concentration.

37. Why is monitoring required for deferasirox (Exjade®) therapy? What are its side effects?

Deferasirox is generally well tolerated, but monitoring for side effects is recommended. The most common side effects of deferasirox include mild, non-progressive increases in the **serum creatinine** (a blood test to measure kidney function) in 34% of patients, and protein in the urine in 19% of patients—findings that basically mean that the kidneys are not working as well as normally would be the case. Gastrointestinal disturbances (nausea, vomiting, diarrhea, and/or abdominal pain) occur in 26% of patients. The gastrointestinal side effects usually depend on the medication dose, typically are mild to moderate, and usually decline with continued therapy. Less common side effects include skin rash, occurring in 7% of patients, which is also usually short-term and mild. However, if gastrointestinal or skin side effects should be moderate to severe, then you should inform your doctor, who will likely hold the drug, then re-start it at a lower dose, gradually increasing the dose as your body tolerates it. Topical or, in some cases, oral steroids may be required for more severe rash. Liver function abnormalities have been observed in 2% of patients, but in most cases, these problems were present before the start of

Serum creatinine

a blood test that measures kidney function.

deferasirox and were most likely related to iron overload in the liver. High-frequency hearing loss and changes in the lens of the eye are rare.

During clinical trials of deferasirox, the drug's effects on iron removal were monitored by a monthly blood test checking the serum ferritin level. Monitoring serum ferritin levels every 1 to 3 months is a reasonable interval to check progress with deferasirox. Monitoring of kidney and liver function is generally performed monthly during the first several months of therapy, with less frequent monitoring over time if kidney and liver function are normal. Ear (audiology) and eye (ophthalmology) testing should be performed before treatment is begun and annually thereafter.

38. Can I take antibiotics to prevent infections if I have a low white cell count?

Using antibiotics to prevent infections when a patient has neutropenia is not standard practice, although some hematologists will use antibiotics in this fashion. Some studies do indicate that certain classes of antibiotics can reduce the incidence of neutropenic fever or infections in patients receiving chemotherapy for blood cancers. However, in such cases, the period of neutropenia is limited to the time of cell count recovery following chemotherapy, usually 3 to 4 weeks. In contrast, neutropenia in patients with MDS can last from months to years. There are no specific studies that support the use of prophylactic antibiotics in MDS patients with neutropenia. However, if an MDS patient with neutropenia has repeated fever or infections, antibiotics could be considered to reduce future infections. One primary concern in using prophylactic antibiotics on a long-term basis is the development of resistance to such antibiotics, as well as the potential for spreading resistant bacteria to other patients.

39. Will I need a catheter or venous access device?

Once a patient is diagnosed with MDS, he or she requires frequent blood draws. The frequency depends on the severity of the disease. Many people do not require a catheter or venous access device at first because most people's veins do not present much problem to technicians taking blood samples. However, if the blood draws are frequent, the veins can become difficult to penetrate; some patients who have particularly narrow veins also may be difficult to collect blood samples from in the first place. In such patients, an access device may be necessary.

A **peripheral venous access device**, also called a peripherally inserted central catheter or PICC, is a line much like a semi-permanent IV inserted into the arm (Figure 5). Inserting the line is a relatively simple outpatient procedure. It is usually done by a physician or specially trained nurse. Chest catheters are inserted below the collarbone and are inserted by a surgeon as an outpatient surgery (Figure 6). Both of these types of catheters extend out of the skin and must be taped up for showering and bathing. Your nurse will teach you how to change the bandage, clean the exit site, and flush fluid through the catheter to keep it clean and free of blood clots.

Peripheral venous access device

a catheter inserted into a peripheral vein for long-term drug therapy or blood monitoring.

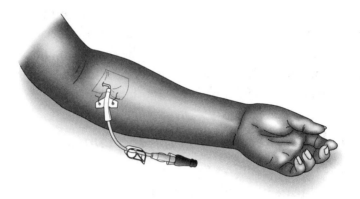

Figure 5   Peripherally inserted catheter device (PICC).

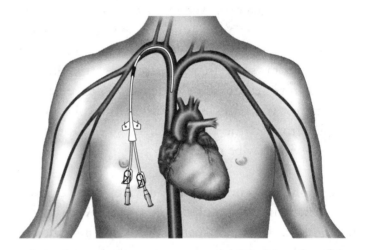

Figure 6   Central venous catheter surgically inserted into a large vein in the chest.

Ports and portacaths are more permanent catheters inserted under the skin, usually as an outpatient surgery. Ports and portacaths are options for patients who will need frequent blood draws, transfusions, and possibly fluids for hydration for the rest of their lives. Because they are located under the skin, they require a nurse to insert a special needle through the skin to access the device. The advantages include easy access for people whose arm veins are difficult to access and having the entire device protected by the skin, so that once the incision from the surgery to insert a port or portacath has healed, the patient can shower or bathe without worry of getting an open site wet. Also, this kind of access device requires flushing less often, which is another advantage.

Any of these access devices can increase your chances of getting an infection. If you get a fever while you have a catheter, you should call your doctor or nurse immediately. You will be instructed as to how to proceed if you get a fever after office hours. If your doctor is not available after hours, you will likely be told to go to the nearest emergency room. If your white blood cell count is low, any infection is an emergency. Any of these devices may need to be removed if you get a serious infection or the device gets a blood clot in or around it. Frequently, the device will be replaced once the problem has resolved.

40. What are hematopoietic growth factors and why are they used?

Hematopoietic growth factors are synthetic versions of proteins made by our own bodies that stimulate red blood cell production and white blood cell production in the bone marrow. They improve the ability of our blood cells to perform their natural functions by increasing the overall cell count in the blood. Of principal importance is the growth factor **erythropoietin (EPO)**, a hormone made by the kidneys that circulates in the blood and travels to the bone marrow to stimulate the growth and survival of developing red blood cells. This growth factor commonly is prescribed for anemia and is the one you have most likely read about

Hematopoietic growth factors

drugs that mimic certain blood proteins to stimulate the production of red or white cells in the bone marrow.

Erythropoietin (EPO)

a kidney hormone that stimulates red blood cell production in the bone marrow.

in the sports pages. For example, cycling or track-and-field athletes have abused EPO, a form of "blood doping," to improve their performance. The goal of the athlete is the same as the goal of the physician who uses them for an anemic patient: to encourage the production of more healthy red cells so that there are more cells bringing oxygen to body tissues—but where the athlete uses it illicitly to get an edge on the competition, an anemic patient needs it simply so that his or her body will function normally. There are two growth factors that stimulate white blood cells: **granulocyte-colony stimulating factor (G-CSF)** and **granulocyte-macrophage colony stimulating factor (GM-CSF)**.

Granulocyte-colony stimulating factor (G-CSF)

a hormone that stimulates white blood cell production.

Granulocyte-macrophage colony stimulating factor (GM-CSF)

a hormone that stimulates production of white blood cells, particularly macrophages.

In MDS, there are two possible situations: either insufficient amounts of these growth factors are made in the body, or the developing white blood cells and red blood cells in the marrow become less responsive to these stimulating growth factors. The rationale for using high doses of these white blood cell and red blood cell growth factor "booster injections" is to artificially stimulate bone marrow production of white blood cells and red blood cells, with the goal of improving neutropenia and anemia, respectively.

41. When should I start using red blood cell growth factor injections?

Although there is no specific hemoglobin or hematocrit value that triggers the use of EPO injections to stimulate red blood cell production, a hemoglobin decrease to around 10 g/dL (a hematocrit value of 30) is often used by hematologists. However, EPO injections may be started at a higher hemoglobin value if it seems that the patient's fatigue or anemia-related symptoms are related to the decreasing red blood cell count, even if the hemoglobin is still about 10 or 11 g/dL. This may be particularly relevant in patients with heart or lung disease who may experience fatigue, shortness of breath, or chest pain at a relatively higher hemoglobin level than patients without these medical problems. Both doctors' evaluation of hemoglobin values and patient symptoms are similarly used to guide the timing of red blood cell transfusions.

42. What is the difference between short- and long-acting red blood cell growth factor injections?

Commercially available EPOs are sold under the trade names Procrit® and Epogen®. These red blood cell growth factor injections are injected into the fat under the skin (usually of the arm), referred to as subcutaneous tissue. In many of the earlier trials of EPO in MDS, the injections were often administered daily, or at least three times weekly. Because of the inconvenience of administering injections so frequently, particularly if a patient's insurance requires the injections to be given in a doctor's office, this is usually no longer done. Instead, the injections are typically administered two or three times weekly. When EPO is dosed three times weekly, a typical dose is 20,000–30,000 units for each injection. When EPO has been studied in MDS patients on a once-weekly administration schedule, red blood cell responses have been observed. Trials directly comparing once-weekly, twice-weekly, and three times per week doses of EPO (to achieve the same cumulative dose) have not been conducted in MDS, so it is unknown whether weekly injections are less effective than more frequent injections. However, since EPO has a relatively short half-life and frequent injections are required to maintain active levels, the current recommendation is two to three times weekly. A longer-acting form of EPO, known as darbepoetin alfa (Aranesp®), has been studied in clinical trials in primarily lower-risk, anemic MDS patients on a once-weekly basis.

43. How long should I try red blood cell growth factor injections? How will I know if they are working for me?

We recommend at least a 6- to 8-week trial of either standard EPO or darbepoetin. If your doctor finds even a minor red blood cell response occurs, you and your physician should consider allowing more time for the injections to elicit a major response, since some studies indicate that higher levels of hemoglobin or decreases in the need for red blood cell transfusions can still occur with more prolonged administration. However, if no red blood cell response is observed after 8 weeks, it is unlikely that continued dosing of EPO will produce a benefit.

Researchers analyzing data from numerous trials have found that the overall response rate to standard EPO in MDS is approximately 20%. This overall response rate reflects a mixture of studies using different doses and schedules of EPO, lower- and higher-risk MDS patients, and different eligibility and response criteria. Several studies have evaluated the predictors of a red blood cell response with EPO treatment. A consistent finding is that patients that have a history of requiring no or relatively few red blood cell transfusions (for example, fewer than 2 units/month) have a better injections in several different diseases or indications, there are several side effects that occur at a similar frequency in both groups. Possible side effects that have been attributed to EPO include increases in blood pressure and a constellation of symptoms at the injection site, such as redness, pain, itching, or swelling. More frequent blood pressure monitoring and withholding of EPO may be required if hypertension (high blood pressure) is noted by your doctor. Other possible symptoms include fever, headaches, nausea, muscle aches or soreness, diarrhea, leg swelling, cough, or chest pain. If a patient is receiving hemodialysis for kidney failure, an increased risk of clot at the vascular access site can occur. Patients are advised to notify their doctor if they have a history of clots in the extremities or lungs, history of high blood pressure or heart disease, stroke, blood disorders such as sickle cell anemia, and if they are pregnant or planning to become pregnant.

Several recent large studies of EPO in patients with solid tumors indicate that EPOs were associated with several adverse consequences if the target hemoglobin was above 12 g/dL. The FDA has now mandated that the prescribing information for EPOs include warnings about the potential risks associated with increasing the hemoglobin above 12 g/dL, specifically:

1. an increase in the chance of heart attack, stroke, heart failure, blood clots, and death;
2. an increase in the growth of a tumor in patients with cancer; and
3. in patients with cancer who have finished planned chemotherapy, an increase in the chance of death regardless of hemoglobin level.

chance of response to EPO. In addition, if you have relatively low levels of EPO in your bloodstream (measured by a blood draw) before you start getting synthetic EPO injections, studies show that you have a better chance of responding to the EPO injections. Conversely, people who have higher EPO levels to begin with are less likely to see any benefit with EPO injections. The reason for this is that the kidneys are making so much EPO already that providing more by injecting a synthetic form of the hormone will likely not affect the bone marrow, which is already highly stimulated by the body's own EPO.

A relatively lower EPO level and history of fewer red blood cell transfusions are similarly useful for predicting response to darbepoetin in the studies of MDS published at the time of this writing.

An important factor that predicts a lower chance of responding to EPO is if a patient has the RARS subtype of MDS, although why this subgroup of MDS patients responds less well to EPO is not well understood. Overall, the chance that a patient with RARS will respond to EPO is less than 10%. However, the addition of a white blood cell–stimulating injection (G-CSF) to EPO can increase the red blood cell response in MDS patients with the RARS subtype (see Question 26).

44. What are the most common side effects of red blood cell growth factor injections?

Red blood cell growth factor injections, either standard or long-acting formulations, are generally very well tolerated. When EPO has been compared to **placebo**

Placebo

an inert s
that has n
body syst
for compa
poses in d

Taken together, these studies included hundreds to thousands of patients with various forms of anemia, but such large-scale studies have not been performed specifically in MDS patients. In addition, no study in MDS has been purposefully designed to answer the questions raised by the solid tumor studies. Currently, no data exist to support the contention that EPOs are associated with decreased survival or increased cardio-vascular related events such as heart attack or stroke in MDS patients. However, it may be prudent practice for hematologists to apply the FDA warning to MDS and use a ceiling level of 12 g/dL for the hemoglobin. If you have concerns about these side effects, discuss them with your doctor.

45. When are white blood cell growth factor injections indicated for MDS?

Synthetic white blood cell growth factor injections con-sist of either granulocyte-colony stimulating factor (G-CSF, also called Neupogen) or granulocyte-macrophage colony stimulating factor (GM-CSF, also called Leukine). Either of these growth factors can be very effective in not only increasing the white blood cell count, but also increasing the subset of important infec-tion-fighting cells called neutrophils. Because of the more difficult side effect profile of GM-CSF, G-CSF is the white blood cell growth factor injection that is favored and commonly used.

The presence of a low white blood cell or neutrophil count alone is not considered a sufficient medical indi-cation to use G-CSF for routine infection prevention. G-CSF should be considered for MDS patients who have both a low neutrophil count and a history of recurrent or resistant infections, or for patients with active neutropenic fever or infection. As discussed in Question 46, G-CSF can also be combined with EPO to treat MDS-related anemia.

46. Why and when are white blood cell growth factor injections combined with red blood cell growth factor injections to help my anemia?

An interesting observation in MDS is that the addition of the white blood cell–stimulating hormone G-CSF to EPO can increase the red blood cell response rate in selected MDS patients. It would seem odd that a white blood cell growth factor injection can help improve the red blood cell count in MDS patients. Although the mechanism(s) for this is not entirely known, G-CSF may work with EPO to prevent the premature death of developing red blood cells in the bone marrow.

In patients with the RARS subtype of MDS who are being considered for hematopoietic growth factor therapy, it is recommended that treatment be initiated with a combination of EPO and G-CSF rather than EPO alone, because of the poor response rate when EPO is used by itself in this patient population. Overall, the red blood cell response rate to EPO + G-CSF is in the range of 30%–40%, compared to less than 10% who respond to EPO alone.

In non-RARS MDS patients who have no or a minimal response to adequate doses of EPO for a 6–8 week trial period, the addition of G-CSF can be considered. The dose of G-CSF recommended by the National

Comprehensive Cancer Network (NCCN) is 1–2 mcg/kg one to three times weekly. For convenience sake, we have typically used a dose of 2.5 mcg/kg twice weekly given on the same days of the EPO injection (e.g., Mondays/Thursdays or Tuesdays/Fridays).

Similar to the experience with EPO, a history of no or fewer red blood cell transfusions and a relatively lower EPO level predict response to the combination of EPO + G-CSF.

47. What are the most common side effects of white blood cell growth factor injections?

Injection of recombinant G-CSF raises its level in the body substantially above the natural levels, so it may produce side effects. A common complaint is bone pain, which is usually mild, but can occur as a more severe ache or discomfort in regions such as the back, pelvis, arms, or legs. Injection site irritation, manifested by redness, itching, or pain, may occur in some patients. Patients may become more tolerant to these symptoms over time. These symptoms stop when the G-CSF injections are completed. Acetaminophen or NSAIDs such as ibuprofen sometimes relieve the bone pain, but as mentioned before, NSAIDs should be avoided if you have a low platelet count (and if you're in doubt about your platelet status, ask your doctor or nurse before taking anything other than acetaminophen).

Less frequent side effects of G-CSF treatment include flu-like symptoms such as fever, chills, and fluid retention, and gastrointestinal symptoms including nausea, vomiting, and diarrhea. A very small number of patients may also develop unpredictable decreases in the platelet count with G-CSF. If this happens, your doctor will likely discontinue G-CSF and begin monitoring of the blood counts to look for recovery of the platelet count.

When using G-CSF, an excessive increase in the white blood cell and/or neutrophil count may occur. In these cases, it is appropriate for the physician to skip one or more doses of G-CSF, and subsequently reduce the amount of medication in later doses.

48. Can white blood cell growth factor injections stimulate the progression of MDS to AML?

If and when MDS changes from a state of lower-risk to higher-risk disease, and then to AML, the percentage of blasts within the marrow increases over time, and there is a potential for G-CSF to stimulate blast growth. Despite concerns that use of G-CSF could stimulate progression of MDS to leukemia, studies of MDS have not shown that this occurs. Nevertheless, in patients with higher-risk MDS, especially those with circulating blasts in the blood or who have increasing bone marrow blasts over time (especially where the blast proportion is greater than 10%), we still recommend caution in the use of G-CSF. If increases in the blood or bone marrow blasts closely follow the use of G-CSF, it should be discontinued. However, it is often challenging to sort out whether the blast increase is related to use of G-CSF or is simply related to progression of the underlying MDS. To help clarify this situation, we recommend that G-CSF be stopped approximately 10–14 days before a bone marrow biopsy is performed so that interpretation of the marrow blast count and the number and morphology of white blood cells is not confused by G-CSF therapy.

49. Are injections available to increase the platelet count?

As of the writing of this book, there are no injections that are specifically FDA-approved for use in MDS to stimulate the platelet count. However, an experimental drug called AMG531, which is given subcutaneously, is currently in early clinical trials in patients with MDS. The drug is being tested both as a single agent and in combination with other drugs, such as 5-azacitidine or decitabine, in patients with intermediate- and higher-risk MDS. Additional experimental medications to improve the platelet count, administered in pill form, are currently being tested in other diseases in which the platelet count is low. It is very likely that these medications will be tested in patients with MDS on an experimental basis in the near future.

In one study, a medication called interleukin-11 (IL-11) was able to increase platelet counts in some patients with MDS. The medication was given to 33 patients with various types of bone marrow failure, including 14 MDS patients. Six of the 14 MDS patients (43%) responded.[9] IL-11 was administered as a relatively low dose in order to decrease side effects. Although generally well tolerated at the lower dose, fatigue, leg swelling, and redness

---

[9]Tsimberidou AM, Giles FJ, Khouri I, et al. Low-dose interleukin-11 in patients with bone marrow failure: update of the M. D. Anderson Cancer Center experience. *Ann Oncol* 2005; 16:139–145.

of the eyes were the more common complaints. In a follow-up study of 32 MDS patients, the platelet count responded in 28% of patients.[10]

50. How is 5q– syndrome different from other forms of MDS?

5q– syndrome refers to a specific subtype of MDS associated with an abnormality of one of the copies of chromosome 5. As discussed in Question 19, a chromosome consists of a short arm, represented by the letter "p," and a long arm, represented by the letter "q." In 5q– syndrome, a specific portion within the long arm of chromosome 5 is missing. The missing segment of the chromosome is denoted by a minus sign "–." Therefore, this subtype of MDS is referred to as 5q– syndrome; in some medical journals, you may also see it written as del(5q) MDS, where "del" is an abbreviation for "deleted," which means absent or missing. 5q– is the most common chromosome abnormality found in MDS, occurring in approximately 10%–15% of patients.

As a subtype of MDS, 5q– syndrome has a relatively favorable prognosis and a relatively low rate of transformation to AML compared to other MDS subtypes. Patients suffer from persistent anemia, the need for repeated red blood cell transfusions, and the potential for iron overload and its associated complications. 5q– syndrome occurs with a slightly higher frequency in women, compared to other MDS subtypes that typically occur more commonly in men.

---

[10]Montero AJ, Estrov Z, Freireich EJ, et al. Phase II study of low-dose interleukin-11 in patients with myelodysplastic syndrome. *Leuk Lymphoma* 2006; 47:2049–2054.

5q– syndrome also may present with unique laboratory or pathologic features in the bone marrow. For example, at the time of diagnosis, some patients with 5q– syndrome often have an increased platelet count, and the bone marrow may show increased numbers of megakaryocytes, the marrow cells that give rise to platelets.

5q– syndrome patients have a prognosis that is similar to, or perhaps slightly better than, other forms of low-risk MDS. However, patients who have additional chromosome abnormalities in addition to 5q–, or who have 5q– with more than 5% blasts in the marrow, have a worse prognosis, including a higher risk of transformation to AML.

51. What is the first-line treatment of 5q– MDS?

Lenalidomide (brand name Revlimid®) is recommended as the first treatment of choice in patients with 5q– MDS. The drug is currently FDA-approved for 5q– MDS patients who depend on blood transfusions to maintain a normal red cell count and who have a low- to intermediate-1 IPSS score. Lenalidomide is considered the first treatment of choice because it has a high rate of red blood cell responses, including substantial improvements in the hemoglobin (often sufficient to allow patients to stop receiving transfusions), in patients receiving regular red blood cell transfusions. In addition, a high percentage of patients with 5q– MDS treated with lenalidomide will develop a **chromosome remission** (Question 52). Despite these encouraging possibilities, you may not be given this drug right away if you have 5q– MDS;

Chromosome remission

a reduction or elimination of cells in which chromosome abnormalities are present.

your doctor will discuss with you if and when treatment with lenalidomide is appropriate. For example, if you only have mild anemia and/or no symptoms, it would be too early to start lenalidomide.

Meredith's comment:

I was very fortunate to be in a clinical trial for lenalidomide, or Revlimid, at Stanford University Medical Center. I responded very well and have been transfusion-free for close to four years.

52. How does lenalidomide affect the blood and chromosomes? How many patients get these benefits from lenalidomide?

In 2006, the results of a study showing how lenalidomide affects MDS patients with the 5q– chromosome abnormality were published.[11] The patients were divided into two groups: some were given 10 mg of the drug daily for the duration of the study, while others alternated between taking the same dose daily for three weeks, then no medication for one week before resuming daily doses for three weeks again. These results were very encouraging: of the 148 patients who participated in the study, 112 (76%) had red blood cell responses. Specifically, 99 patients (67%) no longer needed red blood cell transfusions after 24 weeks of therapy, and 13 patients (9%) had a 50% or greater reduction in the number of transfusions needed. Four patients responded so well, they actually developed an

---

[11]List A, Dewald G, Bennett J, et al. Lenalidomide in the myelodysplastic syndrome with chromosome 5q deletion. *N Engl J Med* 2006; 355:1456–1465.

excessive rise in the hemoglobin to levels above normal. Most importantly, no difference in response was observed between the patients who received continual dosing and those who had on-and-off dosing.

At the time of the study's publication, patients had been followed for an average of 2 years since the start of lenalidomide treatment, and 53 of the 112 responding patients were still transfusion-independent. In 61 of 99 patients (62%) who had responded, freedom from transfusions was still ongoing at 1 year. But what about those patients that *didn't* respond? The study found that there were two factors that lowered a patient's chance of having a red blood cell response: a platelet count less than 100,000/mm^3 and a history of requiring relatively more frequent red blood cell transfusions. It is of interest that when 106 of the original patients had follow-up tests, analysis of their marrow cells found that signs of blood cell dysplasia had disappeared in 38 of these patients.

Lenalidomide also appears to help eliminate cells with chromosomal abnormalities. Among the 85 patients with adequate follow-up chromosome analyses, 62 patients showed improvement in their chromosomes (73%), and 38 of the 85 patients (45%) showed a complete chromosome remission (that is, no abnormal chromosomes were detected). It made little difference if patients had the 5q– chromosome abnormality alone, or had additional chromosome abnormalities; they still showed improvement. The only two factors associated with a lower chance of obtaining a chromosome response were a platelet count of less than 100,000/mm^3 and age of 60 years or less.

In short, the study found that many patients with 5q– syndrome respond very well to lenalidomide, both in terms of an improvement in their red blood cell counts and a decrease (or disappearance) of cells with chromosomal abnormalities. These results led the FDA to approve lenalidomide in December 2005 for transfusion-dependent low and intermediate-1 risk MDS patients.

53. What are the side effects of lenalidomide?

Myelosuppression

a reduction in blood cell counts due to a particular medication.

In the study of 5q– patients, the most common side effect of lenalidomide therapy was **myelosuppression**, a medical term which describes drug-related reduction in the blood counts. A decrease of the neutrophil count to below 1000/mm^3 occurred in 55% of patients, and a reduction of the platelet count to below 25,000/mm^3 occurred in 44% of patients. More severe neutropenia (absolute neutrophil count less than 500/mm^3) was more common in patients on the continuous dosing schedule compared to patients taking lenalidomide for 21 days every 4 weeks. Neutropenic fever occurred in 4% of patients. In most patients, severe myelosuppression occurred within the first 8 weeks of treatment. Other side effects of lenalidomide included itching, rash, diarrhea, and fatigue. These were generally mild to moderate in nature.

One important caution regarding lenalidomide is its possible effects in pregnant women. Lenalidomide is related to the drug thalidomide, which is known to cause severe, life-threatening birth defects. If taken during pregnancy, lenalidomide has the potential to cause birth defects or death to an unborn baby. As such, women who have not yet been through menopause are counseled to use birth control to avoid becoming pregnant while taking lenalidomide.

Because of its potential to cause birth defects, lenalidomide is only available through a special restricted distribution program in which prescribing physicians, through registered pharmacies, are able to dispense the medication. Patients must undergo a survey and telephone interview to assess their eligibility for the drug.

Lenalidomide is also associated with an increased risk of **deep venous thrombosis** (a blood clot in a major blood vessel, usually in the leg) and **pulmonary embolism** (a blood clot in the lung). This increased risk of blood clots with lenalidomide most often happens when it is combined with chemotherapy or steroids, which is a form of treatment used most commonly in patients suffering from a different blood disease called multiple myeloma. A significantly increased risk of blood clots has not been reported with lenalidomide treatment in MDS, where lenalidomide has been used alone.

Deep venous thrombosis

a blood clot in a major vein, usually in the leg, that blocks the vein.

Pulmonary embolism

a blood clot in the lung.

Meredith's comment:

My scalp became extremely itchy during the first or second week of taking Revlimid. I did not know that this was a side-effect, and so tried changing shampoos. That didn't help, but the itchiness eventually disappeared. Bowel movements changed and were poorly formed for the duration of taking the drug.

54. How often will my doctor check my blood counts while I'm on lenalidomide therapy?

Blood count monitoring during lenalidomide treatment has two basic aims: to check whether there have been improvements in the red blood cell count, and to watch for treatment-related decreases in other blood counts, particularly the neutrophils and platelets. The current recommendation is to check a complete blood count weekly during the first 8 weeks of lenalidomide therapy, and then to check complete blood counts at least once a month thereafter. Your doctor's review of the blood counts will form the basis of whether your current dose of lenalidomide is appropriate, or whether the dose needs to be temporarily halted or reduced. Weekly monitoring of blood counts should be considered when lenalidomide is being withheld because of moderate to severe neutropenia or thrombocytopenia so your doctor can assess in a timely manner when the drug can be restarted at a lower dose.

55. What dose of lenalidomide should I be taking for MDS?

The standard starting dose of lenalidomide for 5q– MDS is 10 mg once daily. However, the majority of patients will ultimately undergo dose reduction. In the study of lenalidomide for 5q– MDS mentioned in Question 52, 118 of the 148 (80%) patients in the study required an interruption and/or reduction in the dose of the medication, primarily because of low blood counts. The average time to the first dose reduction was 21 days, and the actual duration of time that the drug was withheld was 22 days. In 50 of the 148 patients (34%), two dose interruptions/reductions were required. The average time interval between the first and second dose reduction was 51 days, and the duration of time of the second dose interruption was 21 days. During the study, the dose could be reduced from 10 mg to 5 mg daily, and subsequently from 5 mg daily to 5 mg every other day. Further studies will need to be performed to determine whether a starting dose of 5 mg daily will be able to reduce the frequency of side effects and the need for dose interruptions/reduction, while maintaining the same degree of effectiveness.

What does this mean for you? It means that while you may start lenalidomide at 10 mg per day, you shouldn't necessarily expect that dose to remain constant for the long term of your treatment. Your doctor may take you off the medication or reduce the dosage, or both, depending on how you respond and whether your blood counts decrease. It also means that your dosage of the medication may change multiple times as your blood counts improve or decrease. If you find the frequent dose changes to be confusing, get into the habit of asking your doctor or nurse at the end of each visit to give you a written instruction sheet for how much lenalidomide you should take. If you are asked to take the medication on alternate days or weeks, use a calendar pill dispenser with days of the week/month to help you make certain you only take it on the correct days.

56. Is lenalidomide effective for other forms of MDS aside from 5q–?

At the time of this writing, there have been some indications that lenalidomide may also help MDS patients without the 5q– chromosome abnormality. In a study of 214 patients with "non-5q– MDS,"[12] 56 (26%) became transfusion-independent, and an additional 36

---

[12]Raza A, Reeves JA, Feldman EJ, et al. Phase II study of lenalidomide in transfusion-dependent, low- and intermediate-1-risk myelodysplastic syndromes with karyotypes other than deletion 5q. *Blood* 2007, in press.

patients (17%) needed transfusions half as often, for a total red blood cell response rate of 43%. For those patients who no longer needed transfusions, it took slightly longer for them to reach that point compared to 5q– patients, and the freedom from transfusions did not last as long—on average, only 41 weeks, where many 5q– patients lasted a year or longer. So although lenalidomide does appear to help some non-5q– patients, it does not work quite as well as it does in the 5q– group. Nevertheless, these data indicate that lenalidomide does have beneficial effects on the red blood cell count and the need for red blood cell transfusions in patients with non-5q– MDS.

Side effects in non-5q– MDS patients are similar to those experienced by 5q– MDS patients: more severe neutropenia and thrombocytopenia occurred at a rate of 25% and 20%, respectively, in the study patients. The rate of dose reduction in non-5q– patients was less than it was in 5q– patients, but the frequency of these side effects are derived from 2 different studies. Mild to moderate diarrhea and fatigue were the most common side effects, occurring in 38% and 29% of patients, respectively.

57. What are 5-azacitidine and decitabine? Am I a candidate for 5-azacitidine or decitabine treatment?

5-azacitidine (brand name Vidaza®) is an anti-cancer drug that has been FDA-approved for all five FAB subtypes of MDS. Decitabine (brand name Dacogen®) is a similar drug that likewise was approved by the FDA for all FAB subtypes of MDS, either newly diagnosed or previously treated, and regardless of whether the MDS is related to prior chemotherapy or radiation (secondary MDS). Decitabine is also specifically approved for IPSS risk groups intermediate-1, intermediate-2, and high. Both drugs are higher-intensity treatments; therefore, they are potentially suitable options for MDS patients with IPSS intermediate-2 to high risk disease in which there is a concern about an increased risk of evolution to AML. In these higher-risk patients, both 5-azacitidine and decitabine are able to delay transformation of MDS to AML. For patients with lower-risk disease who do not have increased marrow blasts, but who do have low blood counts, these agents may be used in an attempt to increase blood counts.

In all cases, the patient and doctor must weigh the potential risks and benefits of using these drugs. This is particularly true in lower-risk patients who may exhibit only anemia. Other drugs such as EPO or darbepoetin should be considered first in a low-risk patient if significant or symptomatic anemia is the only blood count problem, and if the serum EPO level is not too high (that is, a level below 500 U/L; see Questions 40–44). These drugs are generally well tolerated and do not cause reductions in the white blood cells or platelets. However, both 5-azacitidine and decitabine can cause a marked reduction in the blood counts (myelosuppression) for several cycles before a potential increase in the blood cell counts are observed or an improvement in the frequency of red blood cell, or platelet transfusions materializes. Therefore, these drugs may be considered for lower risk patients if other options—such as red blood cell injections for anemia, or lenalidomide for 5q– MDS—are ineffective, or in patients who lose their response to these drugs.

58. How do 5-azacitidine and decitabine work?

One of the reasons that blood cells in MDS fail to mature or differentiate properly is that numerous genes within these cells—genes that normally produce proteins to allow the cells to mature—are turned "off" or made inactive. Some of these genes suppress the development of cancerous cells, and are therefore called **tumor suppressor genes**. These genes can be made inactive by an event called **methylation**, which involves the addition of a molecule called a methyl group to the region of the DNA where the gene is located. This methylation process only takes place when an enzyme called methyltransferase is present. If one or more of these tumor suppressor genes are inactivated by methylation, the absence of activity of the tumor suppressor genes encourages the growth of tumor cells, such as the blasts that may develop when MDS evolves to AML.

This is where 5-azacitidine (Vidaza®) and decitabine (Dacogen®) enter the picture. Both drugs belong to a class of drugs referred to as **hypomethylating agents**, which means that they block the function of methyltransferase (although by different mechanisms), resulting in less methylation of genes. This results in reactivation of tumor suppressor genes, improved cellular maturation, and a decrease or halting of tumor growth.

At relatively higher doses, these drugs act as **cytotoxic** agents, similar to chemotherapy in their ability to kill tumor cells. However, at relatively lower doses, in the range prescribed for MDS, they have the ability to **dif-**

Tumor suppressor genes

particular genes that prevent the development of cancerous cells.

Methylation

a process in which tumor suppressor genes and other types of genes are inactivated by addition of a methyl group to the DNA. Deactivation of tumor suppressor genes can lead to growth of cancerous cells.

Hypomethylating agents

a class of drugs that prevent methylation.

Cytotoxic

refers to substances, such as chemotherapy, that kill cells, particularly fast-growing cells.

ferentiate cells—that is, to cause them to develop from an immature cell to a more mature stage. Therefore, these drugs are also referred to as differentiating therapy.

Differentiate

to cause an immature cell to develop into a mature cell.

59. How are 5-azacitidine and decitabine administered?

5-azacitidine was first approved by the FDA in 2004 based on a phase III trial which compared 5-azacitidine plus best supportive care to best supportive care only. 5-azacitidine was given as a subcutaneous injection at a dose of 75 mg/m^2 seven days in a row every 28 days on an outpatient basis.[13] Each 28 days is considered one cycle of therapy. The drug is given for 1 week followed by 3 weeks of rest. The cycle length of 28 days may be extended to 42 days or longer to allow recovery from low blood counts or other side effects. Because some hospitals do not have treatment centers that are open during the weekends, it has been the practice of some doctors to give the total dose spread out over 5 weekdays, or to have the patient skip the weekend, and come back the following Monday and Tuesday. An IV formulation of 5-azacitidine was approved by the FDA in early 2007.

Decitabine was approved by the FDA in 2006 based on a phase III trial using a continuous IV infusion of 15 mg/m^2 over 3 hours, administered every 8 hours for 3 consecutive days every 6 weeks (each cycle = 6

---

[13]Silverman LR, Demakos EP, Peterson BL, et al. Randomized controlled trial of azacitidine in patients with the myelodysplastic syndrome: a study of the cancer and leukemia group B. *J Clin Oncol* 2002; 20:2429–2440.

weeks).[14] This is administered to patients on an inpatient (hospitalized) basis. An off-label dosing regimen that appears to be effective in preliminary studies from MD Anderson Cancer Center is decitabine infused intravenously at a dose of 20 mg/m^2 over 2 hours daily for 5 consecutive days, on a 28-day cycle.[15] This regimen is more convenient, and is administered on an outpatient basis. It produces a higher complete remission rate (39%) compared to the FDA-approved regimen, but the two dosing schedules have not been compared head-to-head.

If you are on 5-azacitidine or decitabine therapy and your blood counts become very low, particularly severe neutropenia or thrombocytopenia, your doctor will discuss delaying the start of the next cycle and/or dose reduction of these drugs. Your doctor may also consider use of G-CSF and EPO/darbepoetin to try to increase the neutrophil count and red blood cell count, respectively.

Millie's comment:

I have completed two cycles [of 5-azacitidine]. During the time of the treatments my stomach became red, as well as black and blue, and became inflamed. Upon the advice of the nurses I applied several different creams which in time seemed to help. Also during these treatments I experienced

---

[14]Kantarjian H, Issa JP, Rosenfeld CS, et al. Decitabine improves patient outcomes in myelodysplastic syndromes: results of a phase III randomized study. *Cancer* 2007; 106:1794–1803.

[15]Kantarjian H, Oki Y, Garcia-Manero G, et al. Results of a randomized study of 3 schedules of low-dose decitabine in higher-risk myelodysplastic syndrome and chronic myelomonocytic leukemia. *Blood* 2007; 109:52–57.

abdominal cramps. The nurse suggested a medication for this as well. I must add that during this time I felt good in spite of the stomach problems, which have now subsided.

60. How well do these drugs work?

In the studies of 5-azacitidine and decitabine that led to their approval, MDS patients were randomly assigned to one of two groups: the first received the drug along with supportive care, while the second received supportive care alone. As might be expected, in both trials, hematologic and chromosome response rates in the group that only received supportive care were 0%—in other words, nobody who received only supportive care had improvement in their blood counts or chromosome abnormalities.

In the azacitidine trial, the response rates that were reported with FDA approval of the drug included a complete response (CR) rate of 6%, a partial response (PR) rate of 10%, and an overall response rate of 16%. In another analysis of 3 trials of azacitidine (either subcutaneous or intravenous administration), the complete remission rate ranged from 10%–17%, and partial remissions were rare. In comparison, in the decitabine trial, the CR rate was 9%, the PR rate was 8%, and the overall response rate was 17%. Hematologic improvement refers to increases in blood counts without reduction in the percentage of marrow blasts. In the azacitidine trial, the hematologic improvement rate was 36%, compared to 13% in the decitabine trial. In the analysis of all three azacitidine trials mentioned above, the hematologic improvement rate ranged from 23%–36%.

The time to initial response was similar in the two studies. In the decitabine trial, the average time to response was 3.3 months (or 2 cycles) compared to 64 days, or in the beginning of the third month in the azacitidine trial. In responders, the average duration of response was 15 months in the azacitidine trial, and 10.3 months in the decitabine study. However, the caveat is that patients in the decitabine trial were treated for an average of fewer cycles related to the design of the study.

With regard to the chromosome response rate, decitabine was able to produce major cytogenetic responses in 9/26 (35%) of evaluable patients. Data on chromosome responses were not published in the study of 5-azacitidine, and there is currently limited data regarding its benefit in this regard. The effect of both of these drugs on improvement of chromosome abnormalities needs further study.

61. Can 5-azacitidine or decitabine delay the transformation of MDS to AML?

In the studies of 5-azacitidine and decitabine described in Question 60, each treatment was compared to what happens when patients are given only the best available supportive care. These studies showed that using either 5-azacitidine or decitabine *could* delay the development of leukemia—and also prolong the patient's life—in comparison to patients who received only supportive care. For example, in the 5-azacitidine trial of MDS patients of all FAB subtypes, the average time to leukemic transformation or death was 21 months in the 5-azacitidine group compared to 13 months in the best supportive care group. In the decitabine trial, in intermediate-2 or high-risk IPSS patients, the average time to AML or death was 12 months in the decitabine group compared to 6.8

months in the best supportive care group, a statistically significant difference.

5-azacitidine and decitabine are the first non-transplant treatment options that have shown an ability to alter the natural history of MDS—that is, to delay the onset of AML or occurrence of death. For this reason, these drugs may be particularly useful in patients with higher-risk MDS where transformation to AML and shortened life expectancy are important and immediate concerns.

62. What are the side effects of 5-azacitidine and decitabine treatment?

The side effects of 5-azacitidine and decitabine are generally very similar. Myelosuppression, or reduction of blood counts, is the most common, potentially serious side effect of both 5-azacitidine and decitabine. In the decitabine study discussed in prior questions, the rate of severe neutropenia (a neutrophil count <1000/mm^3) was 87%, and the rate of severe thrombocytopenia (platelet count <25,000/mm^3) was 85%. The most commonly reported non-hematologic side effects, irrespective of severity, were fever, nausea, constipation, diarrhea, vomiting, swelling in the legs, and pneumonia.

In the study of patients treated with 5-azacitidine, the rate of severe neutropenia was 58%, and the rate of severe thrombocytopenia was 52%. The most commonly reported non-hematologic side effects, irrespective of severity, were nausea, vomiting, fever, diarrhea, fatigue, injection site redness and pain, and constipation.

63. How will 5-azacitidine or decitabine affect my quality of life?

The studies of 5-azacitidine and decitabine incorporated assessments of quality of life in addition to treatment response.[16,17] Quality of life was judged by different methods, including telephone interviews and questionnaires, with assessments conducted before treatment, at the end of successive cycles, and at the completion of therapy. In comparison to supportive care, patients on both of these drugs said that their quality of life had improved during the course of therapy. One or both of these drugs improved several different aspects of quality of life, including fatigue, physical functioning, psychological distress, and shortness of breath. Since improvement of quality of life is a major goal for both physicians and MDS patients, these results provide an additional rationale for considering 5-azacitidine or decitabine in addition to their potential hematologic benefits.

64. How many cycles of 5-azacitidine or decitabine therapy should I receive?

It is important to realize that both 5-azacitidine and decitabine can take several cycles to show a response; you probably will not feel any immediate results, as disappointing as this might be. We recommend that at

---

[16]Kornblith AB, Herndon JE 2nd, Silverman LR, et al. Impact of azacytidine on the quality of life of patients with myelodysplastic syndrome treated in a randomized phase III trial: a Cancer and Leukemia Group B study. *J Clin Oncol* 2002; 20:2441–2552.

[17]Kantarjian H, Issa JP, Rosenfeld CS, et al. Decitabine improves patient outcomes in myelodysplastic syndromes: results of a phase III randomized study. *Cancer* 2007; 106:1794–1803.

least 3 to 4 cycles be administered before judging the potential benefit of these drugs. Myelosuppression, characterized by worsening neturopenia, anemia, and thrombocytopenia, frequently occurs during the first two cycles. You and your doctor must use patience with these drugs and not jump to the conclusion that the worsening counts are due to progression of your underlying MDS. Use of red blood cell and white blood cell injections may be considered during the first several cycles if neutropenia or anemia worsen. When judging a response, a bone marrow biopsy is performed to assess whether a partial or complete remission has occurred, and whether a cytogenetic response has developed. Evidence for hematologic improvement, a partial or complete remission, improvement in abnormal chromosomes, or at least stability of the disease (particularly if it was previously worsening) is enough evidence to warrant continuing with additional cycles of decitabine or 5-azacitidine. It is recommended that these drugs be continued as long as the patient is deriving clinical benefit and there is no unacceptable toxicity.

65. Which drug is better, 5-azacitidine or decitabine?

Patients often want to know which of the two drugs is the "better" drug, not realizing that there is currently no answer to this question. 5-azacitidine and decitabine are members of the same class of drug—hypomethylating agents—for which the specific mechanisms of action may differ but ultimately may have similar effects on the blood cells in the marrow. In addition, with the approved FDA-approved regimens, they have a similar hematologic response rates and side effect profiles, and both have shown the ability to alter the natural history of MDS by delaying transformation to AML or death. To date, no head-to-head trial of the two drugs has been performed.

Having cited some of the similarities, there are some differences in the ways these two drugs work, and in the clinical trials used to evaluate them. Regarding the latter, different criteria were used in these trials to evaluate the responses to the drug. Secondly, the 5-azacitidine study included a "crossover design," in which patients were allowed to cross over from the supportive care group to the 5-azacitidine group. This crossover design has made it more challenging to interpret some of the study findings. Third, the two studies differed in the number of treatment cycles administered to patients. The average number of cycles of 5-azacitidine administered was 9, but the average number of cycles of decitabine administered was 3. Since it may take 4 or more cycles for a response to emerge, it is possible that some patients on the decitabine trial were undertreated, and that a greater response may have occurred with more treatment cycles. Thus, it isn't really possible to say that either drug is "better" than the other.

Each doctor and patient will need to discuss the relative risks and benefits of each drug before embarking on treatment. The route of administration of the drug (subcutaneous injection for 5-azacitidine, and IV for decitabine) may play a role in which drug to use. However, IV forms of 5-azacitidine are now available, and both medications can be administered on an outpatient basis.

66. How can my health care providers decrease the injection site irritation from 5-azacitidine?

5-azacitidine is given by injection into the subcutaneous, or fatty, tissue located right below the skin. The injection is commonly given under the skin of the abdomen at least two inches from the umbilicus, or belly button area. Redness and pain appearing where the injection was given is the most common reported side effect of 5-azacitidine in clinical trials, where 62% of patients experienced redness and/or irritation at the site. The patients who experienced these side effects reported one or more of the following symptoms: redness, pain, swelling, itching, bruising, and changes in skin color.

To help avoid a reaction at the site of the injection, the injection sites should be rotated. This means giving the injections at a different place each time—new locations should be at least one inch from the previous site. The fatty tissue of the abdomen (at least two inches from the umbilical area), front of the thigh, and back of the upper arm (triceps area) can be used.

Though the doctors who conducted the clinical trials used different treatments to prevent or relieve these symptoms, there have been no formal clinical trials to study these treatments for safety or effectiveness. One possible remedy is applying cool compresses to the area of irritation to numb the pain or burning sensation. You can also take acetaminophen (Tylenol) for the pain if your doctor says it's OK. A cooling cream or ointment such as an aloe vera preparation may give temporary relief; however, we do not recommend using aloe vera taken directly from the plant for MDS patients because it is not sterile, and there is a risk of infection.

67. What is the role of anti-thymocyte globulin and other anti-immune therapy in MDS?

The bone marrow failure that characterizes MDS may result from several different factors. In a minority of cases, the immune system may abnormally attack the developing bone marrow cells. This "autoimmune" attack on the bone marrow results in the death of blood-forming cells, and consequently, low blood counts. In many of these cases, the bone marrow has a low cellularity and can appear empty of cells. Such cases are called hypocellular MDS and resemble a similar bone marrow disorder called aplastic anemia (see Question 17), where the marrow is devoid of precursor red and white blood cells, and megakaryocytes, the cells which give rise to platelets. In other instances, the bone marrow can demonstrate normal cellularity, or a high cellular count.

When autoimmune attack is thought to be contributing to the marrow failure of MDS, anti-immune therapy, usually referred to as **immunosuppressive therapy**, may be a useful treatment approach. This type of treatment is intended to reduce the immune attack on the bone marrow cells. Anti-thymocyte globulin (ATG) has been extensively used in these cases, with variable rates of response. This medication is derived from injecting either a horse or rabbit with human thymus tissue and collecting the antibodies from the animal's blood; the two possible forms are therefore referred to as horse ATG or rabbit ATG. This immune serum is typically administered to

Immuno-suppressive therapy

treatment to suppress the immune system when autoimmune attack on the bone marrow is suspected.

patients as an IV infusion over several hours on 4 or 5 consecutive days in the hospital. Patients are pre-medicated with acetaminophen (Tylenol), diphenydramine (Benadryl), and corticosteroids to reduce the chance of a reaction during the infusion. A small test dose of horse ATG is usually given before the infusion to make sure the patient doesn't have an allergic reaction. In the hospital, intravenous steroids, followed by oral steroids upon discharge, are given to patients to reduce ATG-related side effects known as **serum sickness**. These symptoms may include fever, rash, joint pain, muscle aches, headache, nausea, vomiting, and abdominal pain. Over the course of several weeks, the steroids are tapered off. An oral immunosuppressive medication called cyclosporine is usually started at the time of ATG and is continued for several months. This is a form of maintenance anti-immune therapy. Cyclosporine may also be used alone as a form of immunosuppressive therapy, particularly in patients who may be too frail for ATG treatment or who do not wish to receive ATG. Blood levels of cyclosporine need to be monitored in order to achieve the optimal level. If the blood level is too low or high, the dose may need to be modified. Cyclosporine has potential side effects including headache, nausea, aches in joints, growth of hair where it is not desired, and swelling of the gums. Short-term use of cyclosporine can also cause blood pressure elevation, changes in kidney or liver function, as well as elevation of cholesterol and triglycerides. These functions must be monitored and the dosage lowered if they occur. Because many medications can interact with cyclosporine, it is important to review your medication list with your doctor.

Several factors may predict a higher chance of responding to immunosuppressive therapy including

Serum sickness
flu-like symptoms that are a side effect of horse or rabbit ATG.

younger age, a history of fewer red blood cell transfusions, blood positivity for HLA-DR15 (an immune marker on the surface of cells), and the presence of a PNH clone. This is also a blood test that can be performed in most laboratories.

68. Is there a role for chemotherapy in the treatment of MDS?

If chemotherapy is used in MDS, it is reserved for patients with high-risk disease, which is associated with relatively shortened survival and a higher rate of transformation to AML. The chemotherapy that is administered to patients high-risk MDS is the same type that is given to patients with AML, referred to as intensive chemotherapy. It usually consists of a combination of two intravenous drugs that require the patient to be hospitalized for approximately 1 month. Because chemotherapy causes the blood counts to decrease to very low levels, patients are very prone to life-threatening infections and have an ongoing need for red blood cell and platelet transfusions for 3 weeks or longer in some cases. An additional 2 or 3 cycles of consolidation chemotherapy (chemotherapy to destroy any remaining cancerous cells) may be considered for some patients, or the chemotherapy may be followed by other treatment such as stem cell transplantation for patients in remission who have a matched sibling or unrelated donor.

The MD Anderson Cancer Center in Houston, Texas has accumulated the most experience regarding the treatment of MDS patients with chemotherapy. Similar to patients with AML, older age and poor-risk chromosomes result in poorer patient outcomes (for

Chemotherapy in MDS is reserved for patients with high-risk disease.

example, a lower ability to achieve a remission). Among 510 patients in the MD Anderson analysis, the overall complete response rate was 55%, chemotherapy-related death was 17%, and the 5-year survival rate was only 8%.[18] Different chemotherapy regimens produced similar response and survival rates, but a chemotherapy regimen consisting of the two drugs, topotecan and cytarabine, was associated with a lower rate of treatment-related death.

Because most patients with MDS are older and may have co-existing medical illnesses or poor ability to function, either of which may impair their tolerance of intensive therapy, chemotherapy may not be a suitable option for many patients. A patient's decision to pursue chemotherapy should be considered carefully with his/her hematologist. In recent years, chemotherapy has fallen out of favor as a treatment for MDS. Part of the reason for this is the use of 5-azacitidine and decitabine for higher-risk MDS, which is less intensive, is generally better tolerated, and can delay the transformation of MDS to AML in some patients.

---

[18]Kantarjian H, Beran M, Cortes J, et al. Long-term follow-up results of the combination of topotecan and cytarabine and other intensive chemotherapy regimens in myelodysplastic syndrome. *Cancer* 2006; 106: 1099–1109.

PART FIVE

Stem Cell and Bone Marrow Transplantation

What is stem cell transplantation?

What are the different types of stem cell transplantation?

What factors are considered when evaluating a patient for bone marrow or stem cell transplantation?

More ...

69. What is stem cell transplantation?

Stem cell transplantation is the process in which hematopoietic (blood) stem cells, obtained from a donor, are infused into the patient. Similar to a blood transfusion, the stem cells are infused into the patient's catheter. The infusion is usually well tolerated, but infrequently side effects may occur, such as fever, changes in blood pressure, hives/rash, and shortness of breath. The donor's stem cells travel to the patient's bone marrow, where they settle, self-renew, and divide into developing white blood cells, red blood cells, platelets, and other specialized cells that make up the immune system.

Stem cell transplantation is a really a form of bone marrow rescue. In a **myeloablative** stem cell transplantation, the patient first receives a preparative (or conditioning) regimen, which usually consists of high dose chemotherapy and/or radiation, to kill the existing marrow cells. The purpose of the preparative regimen is to eliminate the cancerous cells in the marrow and to create space in the marrow for the healthy donor stem cells. The donor cells then take over the job of creating new marrow; at this point, it is crucial that the patient get new cells because if no stem cells were re-infused, the patient would likely die from the high dose of chemotherapy administered. After the conditioning regimen and infusion of donor cells, patients have very low blood counts until the donor cells have had time to produce new blood cells, usually several weeks. During this time, patients are at a high risk of infection, require blood product support with red blood cell and platelet transfusions, and need close monitoring of organ function and potential side effects of the transplantation such as graft-versus-host disease (see Questions 70 and 72).

Myeloablative

referring to a treatment designed to kill off the patient's bone marrow cells prior to transplant.

Hematopoietic stem cells are collected from a donor by one of two methods: a bone marrow harvest or a process called **pheresis**. In a bone marrow harvest, the donor has bone marrow collected from the hip bone under general anesthesia in an operating room. Hematopoietic stem cells, which make up a small percentage of the cells within the bone marrow, are then isolated from the bone marrow and stored for transplant. The frequency of bone marrow harvest has decreased dramatically in favor of pheresis, which is a much simpler procedure. In pheresis, the donor is given injections of granulocyte-colony stimulating factor (G-CSF) for several days, which stimulates the release of hematopoietic stem cells from the marrow into the peripheral blood. When sufficient time has passed that doctors believe adequate stem cells have been generated in the bloodstream, a central venous catheter connects the donor's bloodstream to the pheresis machine. Blood from the donor is continuously passed through the machine, and the hematopoietic stem cells are filtered and processed into a collection bag. This process takes several hours and one or more sessions to collect an adequate number of stem cells for the recipient.

Pheresis

a method of collecting hematopoeitic stem cells or other cell types from the blood of a donor.

70. What are the different types of stem cell transplantation?

One way of categorizing stem cell transplantation is by the type of donor used. **Allogeneic** stem cell transplantation refers to donor cells that originate from an individual that is not the patient. In performing an allogeneic transplant, several steps must precede the actual transplant itself. First, a donor must be found in which the **histocompatibility** or **human leukocyte**

Allogeneic

from outside the individual's body; used in reference to transplantation of cells from another person.

Histocompatibility

the extent to which a donor of blood or marrow matches the recipient's HLA type.

Human leukocyte antigen (HLA)

a system of genes encoding proteins that are unique to the individual. These proteins are used by the immune system to recognize native cells from foreign cells.

National Marrow Donor Program (NMDP) Registry

a national database containing HLA profiles of millions of potential donors.

antigen (HLA) type of the donor and patient are the same. Histocompatibility is determined through HLA typing of blood from both the patient and a potential donor (preferably a sibling or close relative) using sophisticated techniques to screen proteins on the surface of blood cells. Do not confuse HLA type with blood type (O+, A+, AB+, and so on). HLA looks at genes on chromosome 6, not a blood factor specifically. Currently, sophisticated, high-resolution DNA typing of 10 HLA genes is used to screen for a full match. The products of these HLA genes are proteins that are recognized by the immune system, allowing our bodies to recognize cells belonging to ourselves from foreign cells.

When HLA typing is performed, the patient and a sibling are first tested to see if they are an HLA match, which is estimated to be a 25% possibility (it is only 100% if they are identical twins). Testing whether a patient and sibling match usually takes no more than 1–2 weeks. If the patient and sibling are not a match, then a search for a matched unrelated donor is conducted. The search for an unrelated donor is conducted by a computer search of the **National Marrow Donor Program (NMDP) Registry**. The Registry lists the HLA type of millions of donors whose blood (or cells from a mouth swab) has been collected and analyzed during blood or bone marrow drives. The NMDP Registry can also tap into international registries, so donors in foreign countries can also be screened. If an initial match is found, it can take several more months to determine whether the unrelated donor and patient are a full match. If a matched sibling or unrelated donor match is found, the donor must be medically cleared to make sure they do not have any diseases that could be transferred to the patient by the infusion of donor cells, and also that the donor can tolerate the process of hematopoietic stem cell pheresis or bone marrow harvest.

Autologous stem cell transplantation refers to use of the patient's own hematopoietic stem cells as a donor source. If a patient is in remission, his or her own hematopoietic stem cells can be collected and stored for use later on, should MDS or AML progress. Collection must be done during a period of remission to reduce the chance that cancerous cells are included in the hematopoietic stem cells that are re-infused into the patient. Autologous transplantation is less commonly used for MDS in the U.S. compared to allogeneic transplantation because of concerns about relapse and its general lack of effectiveness. However, it has been more extensively studied and used as a transplant modality in Europe.

Autologous

from within the individual's body; used in reference to transplantation of cells from oneself.

A third donor source is **umbilical cord blood**. An increasing number of centers are using this approach. Hematopoietic stem cells are collected from the umbilical cords of newborn babies and preserved. A single infant's cord cells contain fewer stem cells than is often required for an adult needing transplantation, so double or "tandem" units of cord blood are often used. Similar to allogeneic transplantation, the cord units must be HLA typed to assess whether they are compatible with the patient. Cord blood registries are available to match prospective donors and patients.

Umbilical cord blood

blood samples collected from the umbilical cords of newborn babies that are stored for later use in stem cell transplantation.

The goal of HLA matching is to find the best match between the patient and a sibling or unrelated donor. The reason for this is that when patients and donors do not have close HLA matches, there is an increased

Graft versus host disease (GVHD)

a condition in which cells within the donor infusion attack the recipient's cells.

Graft-versus-leukemia (GVL)

a phenomenon in which cells within the donor infusion attack the recipient's leukemic cells.

likelihood of severe **graft versus host disease (GVHD)**. In GVHD, the donor's white cells recognize the patient's cells as foreign and attack the patient's tissues/organs. This complication is discussed in more detail in Question 72. As potentially dangerous as this condition is, there is a silver lining: GVHD can correlate with the presence of a **graft-versus-leukemia (GVL)** effect, in which the donor cells also recognize the patient's *leukemia* cells as foreign, mount an attack against them, and potentially contribute to the eradication of the leukemia.

In addition to donor type, transplantation can be categorized according to the intensity of the conditioning regimen: myeloablative, reduced-intensity, and non-myeloablative. Myeloablative transplantation uses high dose chemotherapy with or without radiation to fully wipe out or "ablate" the marrow. This type of transplant has the highest rate of toxic complications and transplant-related death, and is reserved for younger patients (usually those less than 55 years of age) who otherwise have no major medical issues aside from the underlying blood disease. Non-myeloablative transplants use conditioning regimens with either lower doses or less intensive combinations of chemotherapy, radiation, or immunosuppressive therapies. This allows older patients to be considered for these transplants, which sometimes are called 'mini-transplants.' Reduced-intensity conditioning regimens are midway between myeloablative and non-myeloablative transplants in terms of the intensity or doses of chemotherapy or radiation utilized. The experience and long-term follow-up with non-myeloablative and reduced intensity transplants has been limited to approximately the last 10–15 years, so they are still considered investigational.

71. What factors are considered when evaluating a patient for bone marrow or stem cell transplantation?

The same factors used to judge the appropriateness of certain types of medical treatment in MDS are used to evaluate the suitability of transplantation: age, IPSS score, and performance status. Younger patients with higher-risk disease and good overall health are generally considered appropriate candidates for transplantation. In contrast, older patients who have other health problems are not suitable transplant candidates because of higher rates of treatment-related death. The age cut-off for a matched sibling or unrelated donor stem cell transplantation varies between transplant centers, but is usually in the range of 50 to 60 years old. The decision to transplant MDS patients with intermediate-1 risk disease is more challenging, and must be weighed in the context of all clinical issues such as age of the patient, additional health issues, and changes in the pace of the disease. Patients with low-risk disease, regardless of age or overall health, can be treated with less-intensive therapies, and are generally not considered for immediate transplantation. For all patients, the availability of a suitable donor will ultimately determine one's ability to proceed with an allogeneic transplantation. Older patients with a good performance status and higher risk disease who would otherwise not be suitable for standard myeloablative transplants may be candidates for less intensive types of transplantation, such as non-myeloablative and reduced-intensity conditioning protocols.

The availability of a suitable donor will ultimately determine one's ability to proceed with an allogeneic transplantation.

A question that often arises concerns the best timing for transplantation—should it be performed at the time of diagnosis, or at the time of disease progression? A study has shown that in patients with lower-risk MDS (IPSS subgroups low and intermediate-1), it may be best to wait until disease progression; performing transplantation can be more life-threatening to the patient than waiting since his/her chance of dying from MDS is fairly low.[19] In contrast, in patients with higher-risk MDS (IPSS subgroups intermediate-2 and high), the study found that patients were more likely to survive longer if transplant occurred at the time of diagnosis rather than at the time of disease progression, because transplant extended the life of patients who, on average, would have died sooner due to MDS-related disease progression. The decision for intermediate-1 patients is more challenging, as these risks may even out. This study provides some general guidance on the appropriate timing of transplantation if it is considered a reasonable option and the patient has a donor. Ultimately, the decision by the doctor and patient must be tailored according to the individual's situation.

72. What are the potential complications of stem cell transplantation?

There are three basic types of complications from stem cell transplantation: complications related to infection, complications stemming from graft-versus-host disease (discussed briefly in Question 70), and organ toxicity.

---

[19]Cutler CS, Lee SJ, Greenberg P, et al. A decision analysis of allogeneic bone marrow transplantation for the myelodysplastic syndromes: delayed transplantation for low-risk myelodysplasia is associated with improved outcome. *Blood* 2004; 104:579–585.

Because the immune system of the patient is effectively destroyed with myeloablative stem cell transplantation, the patient is very susceptible to infection until the time of recovery of the blood counts. Infections may be related to bacteria, viruses, or fungi. Before transplantation, patients are screened to see whether they have been exposed to certain viruses such as cytomegalovirus or herpes virus. During transplant, these viruses can become reactivated, leading to serious infection. Bone marrow transplant recipients may either use antiviral medications on a prophylactic (preventive) basis to reduce the chance of developing reactivation of these viruses, or only if infection actually occurs. Similarly, antibiotics or anti-fungal medications may be used during the course of treatment if active infection occurs, or on a prophylactic basis.

As discussed in Question 70, graft-versus-host disease (GVHD) is a potential complication of stem cell transplantation that results from donor cells recognizing the patient's cells as foreign. It can range from mild to severe, and in very serious cases can lead to death. GVHD is also classified as **acute** if it occurs within 100 days of the transplant, or **chronic** if it occurs at a later time. Acute GVHD most commonly affects the skin, liver, or gastrointestinal tract, or one or more of these organs at the same time. Chronic GVHD can affect these organs too, but it can also affect other body sites. For example, some patients have persistent symptoms of dry eyes or tightening of the skin, which can substantially affect one's quality of life. Immunosuppressive therapy is used to prevent or reduce acute GVHD, and the doses of these drugs are decreased if minimal or no GVHD occurs. However, if

Acute

occurring within a short time frame.

Chronic

occurring over a long time frame.

acute or chronic GVHD worsens or re-appears, higher doses of drugs may be needed. Drugs used to treat GVHD include prednisone, methotrexate, cyclosporine, and tacrolimus. Short- and long-term immunosuppression can lead to serious side effects, including infection, and can potentially dampen the beneficial graft-versus-leukemia effects of the donor cells (see Question 70). It is for this reason that doctors will try to reduce the dose of the immunosuppressive drugs (or stop them) if GVHD symptoms are very mild or have resolved.

High doses of chemotherapy and/or radiation can have serious side effects on the function of organs such as the liver, kidneys, heart, and lungs. Your doctor will screen the function of these organs before, during, and after the transplant process. A specific type of transplant-related damage to the liver, referred to as veno-occlusive disease, is characterized by fluid-related weight gain, jaundice, and liver function abnormalities. Liver failure and death can occur in some patients. A particular type of lung injury, referred to as pneumonitis, can result from some types of chemotherapy, and heart failure can result from agents such as cyclophosphamide. Bleeding from the bladder can also result, so it is important that patients drink plenty of fluids to "flush" the bladder.

73. What is the chance of my MDS being cured from a stem cell transplant? What is the chance of relapse and death from a transplant?

Substantial information is available on the outcomes of allogeneic transplantation in MDS. Recently, data on approximately 450 MDS patients from the International Bone Marrow Transplant Registry (IBMTR) from 1989–1997[20] were reviewed. The average age of patients was 38 (range 2–64 years), and the MDS subtypes were divided between RA/RARS (40%) and RAEB/RAEB-T (60%). At 3 years of follow-up, disease-free survival was 40%. At this time-point, the relapse rate was 23%, and the rate of treatment-related mortality was 37%. When analyzing all MDS patients together who proceed to HLA-matched sibling allogeneic stem cell transplantation, an overall cure rate of approximately 35%–45% is found.

Patients with a lower percentage of marrow blasts (that is, less than 5%) have better transplant outcomes than patients with a higher percentage of blasts. Similarly, patients with lower IPSS scores have better transplant results than patients with higher IPSS scores. For example, for MDS patients with less than 5% blasts and either HLA-matched related or unrelated donors, 3-year survival rates of 65%–70% have been observed. This is in contrast to patients with more than 5% blasts who are alive and in remission in 35%–45% (related donors) and 25%–30% (unrelated donors) of cases. Improvements in supportive care and donor screening may contribute to better outcomes over time.

Improvements in supportive care and donor screening may contribute to better outcomes over time.

---

[20]Sierra J, Perez WS, Rozman C, et al. Bone marrow transplantation from HLA-identical siblings as treatment for myelodysplasia. *Blood* 2002; 100:1997–2004.

PART SIX

Clinical Trials and Experimental Treatments

What other medications have been evaluated in MDS?

What is an investigational drug?

Am I a candidate for a clinical trial?

More ...

74. What other medications have been evaluated in MDS?

There are many drugs that doctors and researchers have investigated in the hope of finding alternative treatments or supportive care methods. Some have been successful, but others have not, and still others are useful only in specific situations. For example, steroids such as prednisone have no role in the treatment of MDS unless a patient's anemia or thrombocytopenia is thought to be partly related to autoimmune attack on the patient's blood cells. This is the situation in rare cases of MDS associated with a condition named idiopathic thrombocytopenic purpura (ITP), in which the platelet count is low due to immune-mediated destruction of platelets.

The search for effective medications is sometimes a frustrating trial-and-error approach. Some therapies have been tried but have not fulfilled the researchers' expectations, including various types of hormones and drugs that are effective against other forms of cancer. In some situations, experiments of individual drugs may be disappointing, but there is still a potential use for the drug in combination with other drugs. For example, two recent trials that evaluated arsenic trioxide in MDS found that the response rates were relatively low. In addition, its IV route of administration and potential for serious side effects make arsenic trioxide a less attractive therapy for MDS as a single agent. However, future studies will evaluate the role, if any, of arsenic, in combination with other drugs. Still other agents may have encouraging effects, but the side effects are too burdensome. Thalidomide, for example, can produce red blood cell responses in a low proportion of MDS patients, approximately 20%, but the potential side effects of sedation, constipation, rash, and neuropathy, can be difficult to tolerate, particularly in older patients.

Ultimately, patients should understand that researchers use the lessons learned from failures as well as successes to search for drugs that not only are effective in treating the disease, but that are easier for patients to tolerate.

75. What is an investigational drug? How are investigational drugs developed into new medications?

An **investigational drug** refers to a medication that has not received formal drug approval by a regulatory agency. In the United States, the Food and Drug Administration (FDA) is the agency responsible for drug approvals.

The manufacturer or marketer of a drug usually spends years evaluating how the drug works through experiments in their basic research laboratories. Before testing in humans, the drug is assessed for short- and longer-term toxicities and side effects in animals. When a drug is considered a potential candidate for further development, the aim of the drug developer is to collect data to establish that the drug will not expose humans to unreasonable risks in early-stage clinical trials.

In order for an investigational drug to be studied in humans for the first time (or an already approved drug being studied for a different disease than the one it was approved for), the physician(s) responsible for the administration and study of the drug must submit an

Investigational drug

a drug that has not received formal approval from the FDA for use in a particular disease.

investigational new drug (IND) application to the FDA. The IND contains information regarding the preclinical activity of the drug, toxicology studies in animals, manufacturer data regarding the composition, stability, and quality controls used in producing the drug, and information on the investigators, clinical trial, and informed patient consent which will be used to oversee the first administration of the drug in humans. The IND is one means of FDA oversight to protect the human subjects who are exposed to an investigational drug or product for the first time. Once an IND is approved by the FDA, and the clinical trial is approved by the institutional review boards (IRBs) of the participating doctor's hospital, the investigational drug may proceed to testing in humans. The different phases of a clinical trial drug testing before drug approval are described in Question 77.

In some cases, a doctor may prescribe a drug that has already been approved for treatment of another disease if he or she has sufficient data to make its use in another disease seem promising. This is referred to as "off-label" use of a drug, which does not necessitate a patient to be entered into a clinical trial. The difference with an off-label prescription is that the drug is not provided free of charge, as it would often be in a clinical trial, and your health insurance company may only be willing to pay for it if your doctor can make a convincing case for why it may work. Off-label prescription can be considered "investigational" in that the drug has not been approved for that particular usage, but the drug itself usually has an established track record and safety profile for some other disease(s) (it would be unethical for a doctor to prescribe a drug that hasn't been approved for any usage, as there is no way of knowing the side effects or long-term risks).

76. Am I a candidate for a clinical trial?

Whether a patient is a candidate for a clinical trial really only depends on two factors: his or her willingness to participate in a study evaluating an investigational drug, and the availability of a trial to suit the particular treatment needs of a patient. Having said this, a patient usually seeks participation in a clinical trial only after all approved drug options have failed or no longer work, or simply because no effective approved drug is available. In some cases, a drug being studied in a clinical trial may show early and substantial promise. Patients may seek enrollment in the trial despite having had few or no treatments previously because either they cannot, or do not want to wait until the drug becomes approved, which can take several years. This permits early access to a potentially effective drug, which is usually provided at no cost in the setting of a clinical trial.

Being a candidate for a clinical trial does not guarantee that you will get admitted into the clinical trial. Whether you're accepted depends on the specific eligibility requirements of the study, which are referred to as inclusion and exclusion criteria. These criteria usually dictate the types of patients that are allowed to be enrolled (using such factors as stage of disease or functional activity of the patient), the length of time that patients are required to be off prior therapies, and the minimal requirements for functioning of organs such as the liver and kidneys. You must meet all inclusion and exclusion requirements in order to be eligible for the trial unless the sponsor of the study grants an exception.

77. What is the purpose of phase I, phase II, and phase III clinical trials?

When a drug shows promise in the laboratory and/or in treating diseases in animals, the next step is to see how it works in humans. This is done in three steps or phases. Phase I trials, which are generally the first trials in humans, typically enroll 20 to 50 patients (sometimes less or more) who are usually either healthy volunteers or patients with advanced disease for whom no other treatments are available or all other approved drug options have failed. The objectives of phase I studies may be several-fold: 1) to determine the drug's safety and to identify any side effects; 2) to find out how much of the medication can be given before side effects become dangerous or intolerable; and 3) to identify a dose that appears well tolerated for the next phase of testing in humans (referred to as the "recommended phase II dose"). Another common goal of phase I trials is to assess how blood levels of the drug change in patients and how the side effects vary in patients across a range of lower to higher doses. Phase I trials are therefore also referred to as "dose-ranging" or "dose-escalation" studies. The tested range of doses will usually be a fraction of the dose that causes harm in animal testing. Many different study designs exist for evaluating different doses of a drug. Regardless, because the drug is being administered to patients for the first time, subjects are usually monitored very closely by nurses and physicians, and samples of blood, urine, and stool (if appropriate) may be taken repeatedly. Phase I studies may also provide a preliminary signal as to whether the drug works well against the disease being studied. Because the lower doses studied often have no or minimal activity against the disease under evaluation, patients enrolled at these dose levels are usually not expected to derive any benefit from the drug. In this regard, a patient's participation in the trial may be entirely altruistic. In some cases, physicians may allow these patients to receive a higher, potentially active dose at a later time in the study. However, this depends on the particular trial, and some patients may be too sick to wait for the time when the dose is found that shows activity against the disease.

Phase II trials are performed on a larger number of patients, usually from 25–100, but a few hundred patients may be enrolled. Phase II studies are designed to assess the activity of a drug at a specific dose or speci-fied range of doses derived from the phase I trial, and to continue safety evaluations in a larger group of patients. Phase II trials are commonly referred to as "safety and efficacy" studies. Phase II trials are the trials in which researchers most often discover poor activity or toxic side effects, causing the development of that drug to be halted. Phase II trials may sometimes employ a two-stage design. Using statistics, a pre-determined number of patients are enrolled in the first stage. If a certain number of responses are not observed in this first stage of enrolled patients, or if there are an excess number of safety concerns, the trial is terminated early so a larger number of patients will not be unnecessarily exposed to the drug which lacks activity or exhibits poor tolerability.

Phase III studies are performed with a larger number of individuals, usually several hundred to several thou-sand patients, depending on the disease and treatment being studied. The patients are selected randomly to either receive the study drug or be a "control," meaning that they get an alternative treatment with known effects or are given a placebo (usually, the patient, and sometimes the treating physician, do not know what the patient is being given—that is, they are not told which drug is being given). For example, in the case of MDS, for many years the standard of care has been best supportive care, consisting of red blood cell or platelet transfusions and antibiotics for infection. In a phase III trial of a new drug being evaluated in MDS, patients may be randomized to one group, which only receives best supportive care, and some patients would be given the new drug plus best supportive care. If the patients receiving the drug responded significantly better than the ones receiving only best supportive care, doctors would know that the new drug was effective for MDS. On the other hand, if the patients receiving the drug did the same or worse, doctors would know that the drug was either ineffective or exacerbated the disease (and in the latter case, the trial would be ended to avoid doing harm to the patients who received the drug).

Phase III trials can be very expensive and time-consuming trials to design and run. If a new drug is shown to be significantly more effective than the comparison arm, the sponsor/manufacturer of the drug will submit a formal, comprehensive description of the results of the trial and all pre-clinical and clinical data to the FDA (or other agencies in other countries) in order to achieve drug approval. Review of this regulatory submission often takes at least 6 months, but may take more than a year. It is not unusual for some drugs that have an application for approval pending to continue one or more phase III trials. Continuation of phase III trials is typically done for three reasons: first, they serve as a means of providing an effective drug or product to those in need until the time that the drug actually becomes commercially available; second, they can identify other potential situations for which that drug might be useful; and third, they help the manufacturer accumulate additional data about the drug's safety and effectiveness. In the case of MDS, both 5-azacitidine and decitabine were approved based on phase III randomized trials in which both drugs were compared to best supportive care. Interestingly, lenalidomide was approved by the FDA based on a large phase II, single arm study (there was no comparison treatment in the trial), based on its high rate of activity in MDS patients with the 5q– syndrome.

78. What should be mentioned in an informed consent when evaluating whether to enroll in a clinical trial?

An informed consent is a detailed document that is meant to educate the patient about:

- how a clinical trial will be conducted
- which part or parts are experimental
- the risks and benefits of an investigational drug
- the patient's rights
- the alternative treatments available
- what is required of the patient, including all of the periodic testing and examinations required, and for what period of time they will be required
- what testing or medications are paid for by the trial
- who a participant should contact with questions or concerns during or after the trial

- who is responsible for payment of hospitalization or any care needed during or as a result of the clinical trial
- the fact that participation in the clinical trial is voluntary and may be stopped by either the participant (patient) at any time, or the clinical trial investigator (physician) if either feels it is necessary

Informed consent for a clinical trial includes the process of explaining the informed consent document and answering all questions to the patient's satisfaction before the document is signed. The document must be signed by the patient (or the patient's guardian), the person obtaining the consent (usually a nurse or physician), and sometimes an additional witness. It is dated by all parties as well. The patient or guardian always receives a copy of the signed document for their records. During the course of the trial, updated consents that reflect new findings related to the study drug's side effects or changes in the design of the trial may be distributed to the patients to be signed.

Source: Ethics in Medicine, University of Washington School of Medicine website: *http://depts.washington.edu/bioethx/topics/consent.html*

79. Does a clinical trial or my insurance pay for medical expenses while I participate in a clinical trial?

It depends. Some clinical trials are fully funded and pay for all of the patients' medical expenses related to the trial, but more often the treatment is covered in part by the patients' insurance. Medicare typically pays for expenses that are considered part of the routine, standard care for MDS patients. For most clinical trials, the drug being investigated is provided free to the patient, whereas tests and doctor visits that would be considered standard care for a patient with MDS are covered by the patient's insurance. If you are being considered for a clinical trial, it is important to contact your insurance company to find out what expenses they cover while you participate in a clinical trial. In addition, your hematologist's insurance authorization specialist will determine which costs are being paid for by the trial versus insurance, and which costs the patient is required to pay. In some cases, if a patient continues to be treated with an experimental drug on a clinical trial basis, and the drug eventually gets approved, the sponsor of the protocol may no longer provide the drug for free. If this is not specifically mentioned in the consent for the trial, the patient should ask the hematologist about this matter. Because new drugs, hematology lab tests, and procedures can be very expensive (ranging into the thousands of dollars), the patient needs to clarify all expected trial expenses and know who is paying for them before committing to a clinical trial.

PART SEVEN

Managing Your Health

How do I choose a hematologist?

Should I get a second opinion?

What precautions are necessary with a diagnosis of MDS?

More ...

80. How do I choose a hematologist?

Several factors may enter into the decision about which hematologist to choose. How close the office or hospital is to the patient's home, his or her expertise in MDS, word-of-mouth referral, and whether he or she is part of a community (private) practice versus an academic medical center setting may all be factors which play a role in your decision. However, in many cases, your primary care doctor (an internist or family practice physician) will refer you to one of their group's hematologists, who will be authorized to see you under your current insurance plan. This is often the major practical consideration that predetermines which hematologist you first encounter. If you are hospitalized when you are first diagnosed with MDS, the hematologist that you see in the hospital or his/her partner will follow up with you as an outpatient after you leave the hospital. Because hematologists see many blood diseases as part of their practice, an overriding factor that should guide your selection of hematologist is his or her knowledge and experience in treating MDS. Patients should also ask their hematologist how experienced the pathology group is in interpreting marrows from MDS patients.

Sometimes, a referral simply doesn't work for the patient—either the doctor's office is not conveniently located, or the patient and doctor simply don't "mesh" in terms of their personalities. Should you find that you do not wish to continue with the first hematologist you meet—someone you've been referred to, or who handled your case while in the hospital—you can seek out another by several methods. One of the easiest is to go to the American Society of Hematology website and use their "search for a hematologist" function (*www.finda-hematologist.org*). The questions described above should be readily answered by the staff at any prospective physician's office before you make an appointment. Be sure, though, that you take into account the limitations of your insurance when making your choice.

81. Should I get a second opinion?

A second opinion can be useful for many patients. Second opinions are pursued for many reasons: to confirm the diagnosis of MDS, to evaluate the appropriateness of the treatment plan, to consider participating in clinical trials (which may only be available at certain facilities), to establish care with a more local hematologist, or simply dissatisfaction with the interaction you've had with your first hematologist. A second opinion need not mean that you're changing doctors, however; if you and/or your local hematologist wish to seek the advice of another hematologist who has particular expertise in MDS, a second opinion can be very useful in helping you and your preferred doctor to fine-tune your treatment plan. The MDS specialist can work closely with your local hematologist, who would manage the daily aspects of your care. For example, you may obtain laboratory studies from your local doctor's lab every week or every several weeks, and visit the local doctor every month while keeping additional appointments with the MDS expert either on a scheduled basis (for example, every 3–6 months), when changes in your disease course occur, or when changes in treatment are being considered.

A second opinion can be very useful in helping you and your doctor to fine-tune your treatment plan.

Meredith's comment:

Definitely! I brought my records to another doctor for a second opinion, primarily for increasing my knowledge about MDS. A year later I was called by those doctors and asked if I would like to be in a clinical trial for lenalidomide/ Revlimid, because my records had been checked again and they found the 5q– chromosome. So yes, go for a second opinion. You never know what could turn up in the future.

Christine's comments:

I am the kind of patient who wants to get as much information as I can about my medical condition. Having been diagnosed with an illness I had never heard of, I decided to get a second opinion. I asked for a referral to an adult hematologist who could see me for a second opinion. Although I brought copies of relevant parts of my medical record with me, the new hematologist decided to repeat the bone marrow biopsy and chromosome analysis. This doctor confirmed the diagnosis of MDS and the same chromosome abnormality as found with the initial bone marrow biopsy.

Almost a year later, I decided to seek another consultation, this time regarding whether there might be more effective medications than the one I was taking. This decision has turned out to be the most helpful thing I have done for myself because I am now being followed by this doctor. He is on the staff of one of the Centers of Excellence for the treatment of MDS. I am continuing to see my local hematologist for blood counts and physical exams. My local hematologist receives regular written reports from this doctor, as does my medical doctor.

82. Will I continue to see my primary care physician and other specialists while I am being treated for MDS?

Your hematologist and other specialists should keep one another informed about your medical status.

Yes. Evaluation and treatment of your MDS should not prevent you from continuing care with your primary care doctor or other specialists. Your current set of doctors can be valuable allies with your hematologist in addressing your total health care needs. For example, if you are planning to undergo surgery, your hematologist should work with your surgeon to evaluate whether your red blood cell count and platelet count are adequate and whether transfusions are needed for surgery. A low white blood cell count can predispose you to infection, and the need for antibiotics for procedures (for instance, dental work) or surgery should also be discussed in advance. For patients with active coronary artery disease, especially for patients with angina (chest pain), maintaining a hemoglobin level near or above 10 g/dL is often recommended by cardiologists. Your cardiologist and hematologist should work together to optimize your cardiac health in the setting of anemia. Similarly, routine health care screening (such as cholesterol evaluation, mammograms and pap smear screening for women, or routine colonoscopy) should not be ignored just because you have a diagnosis of MDS. Your specialists should copy your hematologist on their notes so he or she is updated about your other medical issues. Conversely, your hematologist should send notes to your primary care doctor and other specialists so they are aware of your latest MDS-related issues.

83. How do I make the most of my visits to the hematologist?

All doctors, including hematologists, are especially appreciative of the patient who can provide a well-outlined history of what symptoms brought them to the doctor. Such a patient who is able to provide this information is referred to as a 'good historian.' You can make the most of the visit by providing a timeline of your complaints, prior doctor visits, treatments, laboratory studies and x-rays, and in particular, any bone marrow reports or slides. If a bone marrow biopsy has

All doctors appreciate a patient who can provide a well-outlined history of what symptoms brought them to the doctor.

already been performed, the referring hematologist may directly send the slides and report to your new consulting hematologist. In some cases, in order to avoid losing the bone marrow slides in the mail or to avoid delays, your referring doctor may ask you to hand carry the slides. Either way, having the bone marrow slides and report available for your appointment with the hematologist is critical. You should also be able to provide a list of your other medical problems, dates of prior surgeries, current medications, drug allergies, family-related medical problems (especially relevant to blood disorders), and your social history, which includes information such as your marital status, use of tobacco, alcohol, or illicit drugs, and your occupation, including exposure to any chemicals or radiation.

84. What are some common causes of anxiety related to the diagnosis of MDS?

As with many medical conditions, anxiety frequently accompanies the initial diagnosis of MDS. As a chronic illness, there is often uncertainty about the course of MDS, and this uncertainty about the future can result in anxiety. In particular, knowing that MDS can sometimes progress to leukemia can understandably provoke anxiety. In many instances, patients do not require any treatment for mild low blood counts, and a watch-and-wait approach is often pursued by the hematologist. This involves checking blood counts on a regular basis, but no treatment. Anxiety may therefore develop in some of these patients because receiving treatment actually provides a sense of control—with treatment, they feel they are doing something to fight the disease, whereas without it they feel powerless. For patients who require treatment, anxiety can develop from the expectation of potential side effects or from actual side effects during treatment. MDS can have unanticipated effects on the emotional, spiritual, and physical aspects of one's life. Dealing with the illness may compromise one's ability to work, place burdens on a spouse or children, and lead to concerns about financial stability.

Anxiety also originates from doctor visits and procedures such as bone marrow biopsies and transfusions. Patients may also come to hematology visits with certain expectations about response to treatment, and if these expectations are not met, or good results are not achieved, anxiety and depression may worsen. The mental and emotional aspects of a patient's illness should be addressed by your hematologist and other doctors with the same attention and care as the physical aspects of MDS. We always encourage patients to talk about these concerns so we can address all quality of life issues.

We encourage patients to talk about their concerns so we can address all quality of life issues.

Meredith's comment:

Some of them are the anxiety and sorrow about having a shortened life span; anxiety for the well-being of my children; iron overload from multiple transfusions and the method(s) of removing the iron; growing weak; looking pale; just not being well.

85. Which health care providers at the hospital and at home can provide help with physical and emotional concerns related to MDS?

The diagnosis of MDS brings with it challenges and concerns. These challenges may differ for individual patients depending on the severity of the disease, what health problems you already had (preexisting conditions), your age, your ability to cope with a life-threatening diagnosis, and the support available to you from your family, friends, and community.

Different health care providers can address different aspects of your care as follows:

- Your hematologist will be available to offer diagnosis, treatment options, and monitoring of the MDS.
- Your primary care physician will continue to be involved with your general care. He or she will continue your health maintenance exams (for example, your yearly physical) and will see you for any illness not related to MDS. He or she will be in close communication with your hematologist and any other specialists you may have.
- You will continue to work with any specialists you were seeing prior to the MDS diagnosis. For example, if you are being cared for by a cardiologist or a diabetes specialist, you will continue to receive that care from the appropriate specialist.
- Nurses at the hospital and your physicians' offices are a valuable source of information about your disease and resources available to you. They will teach you the necessary precautions to take for symptoms of MDS and the symptoms and side effects of the treatments and/or chemotherapy.
- Social workers at the hospital are there to help with a variety of issues. They can frequently help you find lodging near the cancer center or hospital should you choose to travel far from home for a second opinion or treatment. They can guide you in finding possible financial assistance for purchasing medications and advise you regarding programs or services available to help with the cost of

medical treatment or hospitalization. They may be able to direct you to counseling or MDS support groups available in your area. Social workers can also provide and assist you with an Advanced Health Care Directive (see Questions 94–96).

- A nutritionist or dietitian can help you choose a healthy diet or a diet specifically geared to patients with neutropenia. They can also make recommendations of food choices or supplements to use should you lose your appetite.

- Physical therapists can help you regain strength after a long hospitalization or other period of immobilization. They help rehabilitate patients with strengthening exercises.

- Home health care and hospice organizations are available in many communities and offer many services for homebound patients (see Question 97).

- Private hire nurses are also available in many communities. They come into the home and care for patients for pay. A social worker may be able to provide a list of nurses available in your area.

Christine's comments:

At the hospital, the medical staff—the patient's own doctor(s), nurse(s), and the medical social worker—can provide help with physical and emotional concerns related to MDS. It is important to note that these providers can help only if their relationship with the patient is based on trust.

The doctor can answer the patient's questions about his/her diagnosis, symptoms, and the results if there is trust between that doctor and the patient. A nurse can give immediate physical comfort and sometimes can be an advocate translating the patient's concerns to the doctor and other members of the staff.

The social worker in the hospital will immediately learn about the patient's life prior to hospitalization: Who provided emotional support? What are their strengths (i.e., what makes him/her feel good about him- or herself)? This information will assist the patient in dealing with new diagnosis and treatment. The social worker also can help the patient by referring him or her to MDS support systems in the community.

Of course, the patient's relationship with the doctor continues outside of the hospital. Here the need for physical and emotional support may be even greater as the patient's energy is being used up in the demands of living. A patient may also seek emotional support from a psychiatrist.

One of the most supportive organizations outside of the hospital that I have found helpful is the Aplastic Anemia & MDS Foundation. In addition to providing information and support to patients and family members, this organization holds a conference every year at which physicians who specialize in treating patients with bone marrow disease speak. Patients, their families, and other support people are invited to attend these conferences. I have found that one of the main benefits of attending these conferences is meeting other people with MDS. Suddenly it's an okay disease to talk about and there is a mutual understanding of and respect for the struggles. These conferences are held alternately on the east and west coasts. The foundation can be contacted by phone at 1-800-747-2820.

86. What precautions are necessary with a diagnosis of MDS?

Given the potential for low blood counts with MDS, there are special precautions you can take to increase the quality of your life and reduce risks associated with low blood counts.

If your neutrophil count is very low (especially below 500/mm^3), you are at a higher risk of getting an infection. Moreover, infections that used to be more of an inconvenience, like a cold or infected cut, can quickly become life threatening. Limiting the number of sick people you encounter is one important way to decrease your chances of getting an infection. Ask your friends and family to stay away while they have a cold or other illnesses. If your white blood cell count is low, avoid crowded places like movie theaters, grocery stores, and restaurants. Wash your hands frequently and carry a waterless hand cleaner with you when you go out. Use your waterless hand cleaner after touching door handles, hand rails, and other people's hands. Pets such as birds, cats, and dogs carry bacteria and viruses that may not be a problem for people with a normal white blood cell counts, but could become a hazard to your health. Arrange for someone else to clean your bird's cage, clean the cat's box, and pick up after your dog if your white blood cell is low. Also, you should avoid gardening because of the possibility of exposure to fungal spores, which may become the source of fungal infections of the lung. If you live on a ranch or a farm with animals, talk to your doctor or nurse about how to avoid infectious materials you may encounter. Avoid any stagnant water such as that found in flower vases and ponds. Cook your food well, and avoid food that has been exposed to air, like that found at delis and food counters. Check your temperature if you have any symptoms of an infection like a cough or sore throat, chills, burning with urination, a cut that becomes inflamed, or even if you just "feel strange." Report a temperature over 100.5° to your doctor or nurse immediately.

A neutropenic diet is recommended for MDS or other patients with neutropenia. Foods have both good and bad bacteria; however, while healthy individuals can easily deal with the bad bacteria, this is not the case with neutropenic patients, whose bodies have reduced immune function.

Table 8 shows which foods are allowed and which should be avoided during the period of neutropenia.

87. What MDS-related issues should be addressed if I see my dentist or have surgery planned?

Patients with MDS should contact their hematologist before scheduling dental procedures or surgeries. Because neutropenia or thrombocytopenia can develop during the course of MDS, you could be at risk for serious infection or excessive bleeding during or after dental procedures or surgery. Your hematologist should work with your dentist or surgeon to decide whether you need antibiotics to prevent infection, or whether one or more platelet transfusions or additional medications might help to reduce the risk of bleeding. If inpatient or outpatient surgery is required, ask your hematologist whether the risk of a procedure or surgery outweighs the potential benefits. If this is the case, your physician will tell you the concerns and discuss the alternatives. For example, if you were to undergo an elective dental procedure, such as routine teeth cleaning, with a very low platelet count (that is, below 20,000/mm^3), the potential risk of substantial bleeding would likely outweigh potential benefits.

88. Will I need to be hospitalized for my MDS?

There may be times when you need to be hospitalized for your MDS. The most common reason for being hospitalized is due to fever during occasions when you

TABLE 8 Neutropenic Diet

The following guidelines are general and not complete. Ask your own doctor or nurse before you eat or drink something if you are not sure that it is safe for you.

General Guidelines: Avoid uncooked foods, any foods that have set at room temperature for a period of time, and foods that contain live bacterial cultures. Clean all cooking utensils and surfaces such as countertops and cutting boards with hot soapy water. The person preparing the food must wash their hands frequently with warm water and soap. Do not leave food at room temperature: keep hot food hot and cold food cold.

Foods to Avoid	Acceptable Alternatives
Any raw meat or cold processed meats, such as lox	Well-cooked meats
Ground meat that is not well done	Ground meat that is well cooked
Raw eggs or anything with raw eggs, such as egg-nog	Well-cooked eggs
Raw fruits or frozen fruits	Cooked or canned fruits; Frozen fruits are acceptable only after they are well cooked. Bananas, oranges, and melons are acceptable while raw if someone other than the patient peels the fruit and it is eaten immediately.
Raw vegetables, salads, or frozen vegetables	Cooked or canned vegetables; frozen vegetables are acceptable only after they are well cooked.
Sushi, including cooked sushi ingredients prepared in the same place where raw food is prepared	Cooked foods
Dried fruits or vegetables; many dried fruits and vegetables are made from raw foods and still carry bacteria	Cooked foods
Deli foods	Foods prepared in your own home and properly refrigerated
Cheeses and yogurt made with live cultures or molds; raw milk or cream	Pasteurized milk products that do not have live cultures or molds
Products from bakeries that have sat open at room temperature and are unpackaged	Biscuits, pancakes, and other baked products made at home and eaten right away; commercially packaged breads; cooked rice and pasta
Raw spices or herbs, including herbal medicines	Spices that are well cooked by adding them to the food before it is cooked
Uncooked teas such as sun tea, or any other tea before it is boiled	Use packaged tea bags and boil the tea after it is made.
Well water, natural spring water	Most tap water from central sources and distilled water, bottled beverages
Raw nuts, raw honey	Nuts roasted after being shelled; cooked or pasteurized honey

Sources:

1. Hope Cancer Institute: *http://www.hopecancerinstitute.com/patient_information.htm*

2. University of Pittsburgh Medical Center: *http://patienteducation.upmc.com/pdf/NeutropenicDiet/pdf*

Neutropenic fever

a fever occurring in a patient who has a low neutrophil or white cell count.

have a low neutrophil or white blood cell count. Hematologists refer to this as **neutropenic fever**. This is considered a medically urgent situation because serious and potentially fatal infections can develop in patients who do not have enough white blood cells (especially neutrophils) to fight bacteria or other infections. In these cases, patients will be admitted for a thorough work-up in order to identify the source of the infection. Such tests will include blood cultures drawn from a vein and/or catheter, chest x-ray, urinalysis and culture, and sometimes, stool studies. Another reason for hospitalization would be to control persistent bleeding because of a low platelet count (severe thrombocytopenia). In some cases, patients who have severe anemia and require several units of red blood cells may be admitted to the hospital to complete these transfusions over 1 or 2 days. Finally, some treatments for MDS may require a hospital stay. For example, decitabine is a drug for MDS that may be given every 8 hours over 3 days in a hospital setting.

Some hematologists work with outpatient infusion treatment areas, which are facilities that can administer transfusions and intravenous antibiotics or other medications. These treatment areas can be very helpful in avoiding hospitalizations for standard transfusions or intravenous medications. It is worthwhile to ask your hematologist if such a facility is available in your area.

89. Can I continue taking my usual medications?

When you see your hematologist, always bring all of your medicine bottles with you so that you can update your doctor about which medications you are taking. We suggest bringing the bottles because then you do not have to try to recall dosages and schedules, particularly if you're taking many different medications. You should report all prescription and over the counter medications, as well as vitamins or herbal supplements. It is important that you mention *everything* because some supplements or medications can block the function of the bone marrow, resulting in decreased blood counts, so it is important to ask your doctor about new medications or supplements before starting them. Conversely, if you have already started new medications without notifying your hematologist, and your blood counts start worsening, all medications or supplements on your medication list should be reviewed to evaluate whether they can be contributing to the decreasing blood values. For patients being evaluated by hematologists for the first time because a possible MDS diagnosis is still under investigation, it is particularly important to evaluate whether the medications themselves could be causing the low blood counts.

For MDS patients on clinical trials, certain experimental drugs may not be compatible with medications or vitamins. The hematologist or nurse conducting the clinical study should inform the patient concerning which medications are acceptable and which are not. In addition, even if certain medications are permitted, they may only be allowed to be taken at a certain time frame relative to the MDS clinical trial drug (for example, 2 hours before or after).

90. Should I take vitamins or herbal supplements to help my MDS?

Basic vitamin supplements (such as a daily multivitamin) are not likely to either improve or worsen the course of a patient's MDS. However, the patient's treating hematologist should review the vitamins that are being taken by the patient because some may have negative effects on the blood counts. We recommend that herbal supplements be avoided because supplements are not regulated by the Food and Drug Administration, so their actual ingredient content may not be known, and often there is little or no scientific data as to how the herbs affect bone marrow and blood cells. We have treated patients with MDS and other blood diseases in whom blood counts worsened because the patients took herbs or herb-containing remedies. Stopping the herbs resulted in blood count improvement.

Herbal supplements are not regulated, so their actual ingredients may not be known.

The need for vitamins and iron differs from person to person. MDS patients who have chronic anemia and require frequent blood transfusions often suffer from iron overload (see Question 35). Each unit of blood contains approximately 200–250 mg of iron. In these cases, taking extra sources of iron by mouth can be harmful, so if you wish to take a multivitamin, use a multivitamin formulated without iron. This may seem strange since most people equate anemia with iron deficiency, but in MDS, it isn't the iron that's missing, it's the red blood cells themselves, so taking iron supplements doesn't help and is actually dangerous (particularly if iron overload is already occurring). In some cases, however, iron deficiency exists in addition to MDS, and if that happens, there may be a benefit to taking iron. You have no way of knowing which is the case unless your doctor checks your level of body iron, so consult with him or her to help you decide whether iron supplementation is a beneficial or harmful option.

91. Can I still exercise with a diagnosis of MDS?

Your ability to exercise will be guided by your symptoms. For example, if your MDS is causing anemia, it may be difficult to undertake cardiovascular exercise such as walking or running. Patients typically feel increasingly weak when their next set of red blood cell transfusions approaches. Red blood cell transfusions can make patients feel stronger, feel less short of breath, and permit greater exercise tolerance. A low platelet count can cause bruising or bleeding. Exercising with heavy weights is not recommended with very low platelet counts (generally less than $50,000/mm^3$) because it may increase the risk of skin, joint, or muscle bleeding. Every patient should set his or her own pace of exercise depending on current symptoms. Since MDS is a chronic illness, exercise is always encouraged for the overall health of the patient and may have long-term benefits, such as improvement of cardiovascular health. However, exercise will not improve blood count problems specifically related to MDS.

Every patient should set his or her own pace of exercise depending on current symptoms.

92. For men and for women of childbearing age, will certain treatments cause sterility?

Some cancer treatments, including chemotherapy, radiation, and bone marrow transplant, can cause temporary or permanent sterility. If having a child is a concern for you, discuss the possibility of sterility resulting from the particular treatment you are considering with your physician. Men have the option of banking sperm before starting treatment. Banked sperm may be used as an option for a man to father his own children in the future even if his treatment makes him permanently sterile.

For women undergoing cancer treatment, the process of storing fertilized eggs for future use may be available. This is called embryo cryopreservation, and it involves surgically removing the ova (eggs) from the women and fertilizing them with sperm. The sperm may be from her husband or partner. If she is not married or not in a permanent relationship with a man, donated sperm from a sperm bank may be used. The embryos are then frozen for future use.

Embryo cryopreservation takes time and may mean delaying therapy. If it is something you are considering and treatment is not required immediately, you should look into doing it soon rather than waiting. If you need to start treatment right away, it may not be advisable to delay treatment for the time it takes to collect the ova for the embryo cryopreservation process. Other options are still experimental and may be available as proven alternatives in the future.

It is important to note that there may be expenses associated with sperm banking and embryo cryopreservation that likely will not be covered by insurance. Be certain that you know all of the financial considerations before you move forward with either option.

Sources: Lee SJ, Schover LR, Partridge AH, et al. American Society of Clinical Oncology recommendations on fertility preservation in cancer patients. *J Clin Oncol* 2006; 24:1–15, and http://www.guideline.gov/. Enter search term: fertility.

93. Are there organizations to help me pay for expenses related to my treatment?

Treatment-related expenses can relate to various issues: cost of MDS-related therapy and related medications, inpatient and outpatient costs related to doctor visits and procedures, and travel-related expenses such as gas, local lodging, etc. Before the patient embarks on a medical treatment plan, he or she should discuss with the insurance company and the doctor's insurance authorization official which costs will be covered and what potential co-pays or deductibles will be charged to the patient.

In some cases, if patients can demonstrate financial need, the manufacturer of a drug may be able to pay a portion of the cost of a medical treatment through their patient assistance program. A doctor's nurse or case manager can assist with this process by contacting a representative from the drug company.

If travel or lodging expenses become difficult to pay for, certain organizations may be able to refund costs. For example, in selected cases, the Leukemia and Lymphoma Society (listed in the Appendix) may be able to reimburse a portion of travel costs if financial need is demonstrated.

In some instances, making use of Social Security Disability Insurance (SSDI) may be an option. A person under the age of 65 qualifies for SSDI if he or she has a condition that is expected to last at least 12 months or result in death and that prevents him or her from engaging in any substantial gainful work. The person must also have worked 5 out of the last 10 years and be able to provide medical proof verifying the inability to work. There is a list of Social Security disability impairment criteria, broken down by specific conditions, on the Social Security Administration website (see Appendix).

94. What is an Advanced Directive?

The best person to make decisions regarding your medical care is you. Patients have the right to make their own decisions about how aggressive their treatment and care should be. Unfortunately, there may come a time when you are not mentally or physically able to express your wishes.

An Advanced Directive is a legal document that spells out your wishes regarding end-of-life care. It allows you to answer some specific questions to guide your health care providers and family to carry out your wishes in the event that you are no longer able to communicate or no longer able to make good decisions. It also allows you to name someone to speak for you in matters of medical care if there comes a time when you can not. An Advanced Directive commonly includes a Living Will (see Question 95) and a Power of Attorney (see Question 96).

This document can usually be obtained from a social worker at the hospital. It is a legal form and each state has a specific form. You can also access and download the Advanced Health Care Directive form for use in your state on the National Hospice and Palliative Care Organization (NHPCO) website: *www.nhpco.org*. The NHPCO provides examples of advance directives, living wills, and power of health care attorney appointment forms for each state and the District of Columbia. Your signature must be witnessed or notarized to be legal.

Having an Advance Health Care Directive in place before it is needed helps to ensure that your wishes will be carried out when you are no longer able to express your desires. It also relieves the family of making difficult decisions in a stressful situation.

Source: National Hospice and Palliative Care Organization website: *www.nhpco.org*

95. What is a living will?

When a loved one becomes ill, it can be a very emotional time for the family. The responsibility of deciding whether to continue life support or allow a family member to die peacefully can be overwhelming. Frequently, individual family members disagree on what is best. A living will is a legal document that gives direction to health care providers and family members when the patient is no longer able to express his or her own wishes. It states the patient's wishes to continue or withdraw life support when there is no longer hope of recovery. It can address the question of whether or not to revive the patient when the heart stops, whether the patient accepts or rejects the idea of continuing life with an artificial breathing machine or respirator, or if the patient wants to be fed by a feeding tube.

Creating a living will can be difficult, but the benefit it offers is tremendous. It prevents conflict within your family during a difficult time and can ensure that there are no misunderstandings by your health care providers as to what kind of measures are acceptable once all hope of recovery is gone.

Source: National Hospice and Palliative Care Organization website: *www.nhpco.org*

96. *What is a Power of Attorney?*

A Power of Attorney is a document in which you appoint someone else to act on your behalf. It can start immediately, or you can specify to have it start when you are no longer able to make your own decisions. A Power of Attorney does not designate someone to make medical decisions for you. For that, you will want a Medical Power of Attorney. If you decide to have a Medical Power of Attorney, discuss the decision with the person you would like to designate. It is important to discuss your wishes with this person and find out if he or she is comfortable with the responsibility of making medical decisions for you if you are not able to.

The person you appoint to make your health care decisions is called your Health Care Agent (or Health Care Proxy). This person must be an adult and may be a family member, spouse, friend, or other adult. You may not appoint your health care provider or an operator or employee of the health care facility or residential care facility where you receive care. If the person you choose to be your Health Care Agent is your relative or coworker and is also an employee of whatever facility provides your care, he or she may be an exception to this rule.

Your Health Care Agent will be the person to consent to or decline medical care, tests, surgeries, and cardiopulmonary resuscitation on your behalf if you are unable to do so. This person may choose a doctor for you, sign to release your medical information, and sign to donate your organs. You can write a statement to include in your Advanced Health Care Directive to limit this authority if you wish.

Source: National Hospice and Palliative Care Organization website: *www.nhpco.org*

97. What is hospice care? How do I choose a hospice program?

Hospice care is end-of-life care with the purpose of caring for the individual and their family without any goal of cure. It is a way of treating the patient, and the symptoms of the disease, without treating the disease itself. The focus is on the patent and the patient's family. It includes a team of caregivers trained to provide a gentle approach to supportive care, including the physical care of the patient and the emotional and spiritual care of the patient and family.

Hospice care is usually provided in the patient's home. However, there are some facilities that provide either long-term hospice care to the patient or short-term care, called respite care, designed to provide a break for the family or caregiver. It may be part of a larger facility, like a private hospital or a Veteran's Affairs Hospital, or it could be a small, private home providing care for individual patients. Your health care provider or social worker can direct you to the available resources.

A hospice team will usually include doctors, nurses, social workers, physical therapists, counselors, and volunteers. Your primary care physician or hematologist may or may not work with the medical director of the hospice to make decisions concerning your care. Remember that this is a shift of focus from cure to gentle end-of-life care, and the hospice team is usually most experienced in providing this kind of care.

The first hospice visit is designed to acquaint the patient and family with services provided by the hospice team, and to assess the current needs of the patient and family. During this visit, the goals and philosophy of hospice care are discussed. This is a time for the patient to decide, with their family, whether or not it is time to actually start the hospice care. Sometimes a patient will decide that he or she may want hospice care in the future, but the time is not yet right. If the patient is ready to start, the first visit will include assessing the home and making recommendations for certain equipment that will be helpful for the patient and caregivers.

When the patient is ready for hospice, a schedule of visits will be determined. During these visits, the various members of the hospice team will come to reassess the patient and family and provide care and direction. They may prescribe pain medication or other medications to provide comfort to the patient. They may provide emotional support and counseling to the patient and family. The goal of the hospice team is to best support the patient and family during the last few months of life and through the death of the patient. They are on call 24 hours a day and will come to be with the family to provide comfort and direction as the patient dies. They may also make a visit after the patient dies to visit the family and give direction regarding closure and grief counseling.

When choosing a hospice program, first start with your insurance provider. Ask if they are contracted with specific hospice programs in your area. Most insurance companies, including Medicare and Medicaid, provide some hospice coverage. When you have a list of covered providers in your area, ask your health care provider and social worker if they have experience with each provider. You can frequently read about providers on their websites and conduct interviews by phone or in person. Making your choice early will alleviate stress for you and your family later if hospice care becomes necessary.

Source: The Hospice website: *www.hospicenet.org,* and the Caring Connections website: *www.caringinfo.org*

Making your choice of hospice provider early will alleviate stress for you and your family later.

98. What is the NCCN, and how do I access their guidelines for MDS? Are there other reliable Internet resources?

The National Comprehensive Cancer Network (NCCN) is a nonprofit organization of 21 of the top cancer centers in the United States with the goal of improving the quality of care and treatment for cancer patients and supporting the research needed to attain these goals. It is a valuable source of information on treatments for MDS for physicians as well as symptom management for patients. It provides guidelines for the treatment of many cancers, including MDS. These guidelines are updated at least yearly by a panel of expert physicians from the NCCN Member Institutions.

You can access the NCCN website for more information (see the Appendix) and to order free publications on symptom management including cancer pain, fever and neutropenia (low white blood cell count), nausea and vomiting, distress (feelings and emotions such as sadness or anxiety), and advanced cancer and palliative care. These resources are available in English and Spanish.

The website gives comprehensive information about the physicians and resources available at each of the 21 NCCN Organizations. It provides a map of the United States with each of the NCCN Cancer Centers represented. It also gives website links to each so you can find out referral and contact information.

There are also a number of good general information websites. The Myelodysplastic Syndromes Foundation is a valuable resource for both physicians and patients.

The Aplastic Anemia and MDS International Foundation, Inc. is also an excellent resource for patient assistance; it provides educational materials, peer support, and medical information on MDS and related diseases. Websites and other contact information for both of these organizations are available in the Appendix.

FDA-approved drugs frequently have educational websites designed to assist patients in better understanding the disease and how the drugs work. A number of these are available for drugs used in MDS, including:

- Lenalidomide (Revlimid): www.revlimid.com
- 5-Azacitidine (Vidaza): www.vidaza.com
- Decitabine (Dacogen): www.dacogen.com
- Deferasirox (Exjade): www.exjade.com

You can also learn about clinical trials of new drugs or new drug protocols by accessing the National Institutes of Health (NIH) website, which is the most comprehensive source for available clinical trials in MDS and other diseases. The website user is required to enter terms to conduct the search for the information of interest to the patient. Information on trials is provided including the rationale for the trial, whether it is still recruiting, eligibility criteria, and contact information. The website and other contact information are listed in the Appendix.

99. What are future directions in MDS research and treatment?

In just the last 10 years, laboratory and clinical research in MDS have exploded. Before 2004, there were no approved drugs for MDS; within the last 4 years, four new drugs have been approved by the FDA for use in the disease: 5-azacitidine (Vidaza), lenalidomide (Revlimid), decitabine (Dacogen), and deferasirox (Exjade). Because MDS arises from multiple abnormalities within the bone marrow, drugs with different mechanisms of action are being investigated to treat it. These medications are first being explored in clinical trials as single agents, and are subsequently being evaluated in combination with other drugs to determine their safety profile and effectiveness. For example, a new class of drugs, referred to as histone deacetylase inhibitors, are currently being tested in clinical trials. These agents can stimulate immature blood cells to differentiate into more mature blood cells. One histone deacetylase inhibitor, named MS-275, is being evaluated in combination with 5-azacitidine as part of a large Eastern Cooperative Oncology Group (ECOG) trial in patients with MDS and AML.

The study of drugs that can increase the platelet count is an active area of investigation. Similar to the use of red blood cell injections (that is, EPO, darbepoetin) and white blood cell injections (G-CSF) that stimulate red blood cell and white blood cell production, respectively, the researchers in this field hope to find a drug that can stimulate the platelet count in MDS patients who suffer from severe thrombocytopenia and/or bleeding.

Clinical trials are of critical importance in making progress in the treatment of MDS. Therefore, patient willingness to participate in such trials and to donate blood or bone marrow for research purposes remains a high priority in the future. With an increasing number of sophisticated research tools that can evaluate mutations in DNA, looking in particular at the comparative patterns of DNA and proteins in both MDS patients and healthy individuals, this is an exciting time in the field of MDS research.

Patient willingness to participate in clinical trials and to donate blood or bone marrow for research purposes remains a high priority in the future.

100. Where can I find more information about MDS?

The Appendix that follows includes a list of resources that MDS patients may find useful.

Appendix

American Cancer Society (ACS)

www.cancer.org
1599 Clifton Road
Atlanta, GA 30329
Phone: 800-ACS-2345 (800-227-2345)

American Medical Association (AMA)

www.ama-assn.org
515 N. State Street
Chicago, IL 60610
Phone: 800-621-8335

American Society of Clinical Oncology (ASCO)

www.asco.org
1900 Duke Street, Suite 200
Alexandria, VA 22314
Phone: 703-299-0150
Fax: 703-299-1044
E-mail: *asco@asco.org*

American Society of Hematology (ASH)

www.hematology.org
1900 M Street NW, Suite 200
Washington, DC 20036
Phone: 202-776-0544
Fax: 202-776-0545

Aplastic Anemia & MDS International Foundation, Inc. (AA&MDSIF)
www.aamds.org
P.O. Box 310
Churchton, MD 20733
Phone: 800-747-2820
410-867-0242
Fax: 410-867-0240

Blood and Marrow Transplant Information Network (BMT InfoNet)
www.bmtinfonet.org
2310 Skokie Valley Road, Suite 104
Highland Park, IL 60035
Phone: 847-433-3313
Toll-free: 888-597-7674

The Bone Marrow Foundation
www.bonemarrow.org
70 East 55th Street, 20th floor
New York, NY 10022
Phone: 800-365-1336

Cancer Care, Inc.
www.cancercare.org
275 7th Avenue
New York, NY 10001
Phone: 800-813-HOPE (800-813-4637)
212-712-8400 (Administration)
212-712-8080 (Services)
Fax: 212-712-8495
E-mail: *injo@cancercare.org*

Cancer Hope Network
www.cancerhopenetwork.org
Phone: 877-HOPENET (877-467-3638)

Cancer Research Institute
www.cancerresearch.org
681 Fifth Avenue
New York, NY 10022
Phone: 800-99-CANCER (800-992-2623)

Cancer Symptoms.Org
www.cancersymptoms.org

Centers for Disease Control and Prevention (CDC)
www.cdc.gov
1600 Clifton Road
Atlanta, GA 30333
Phone: 404-639-3534
Toll-free: 800-311-3435

Centers for Medicare and Medicaid Services (CMS)
www.cms.hhs.gov

Health Insurance Association of America (HIAA)
www.hiaa.org
555 13th Street NW, Suite 600
East Washington, DC 20004-1109
Phone: 202-824-1600

Health Resources and Services Administration (HRSA)
www.hrsa.gov
Hill-Burton Program
U.S. Department of Health and Human Services, Parklawn
Building
5600 Fishers Lane
Rockville, MD 20857
Phone: 301-443-5656
Toll-free: 800-638-0742
800-492-0359 (if calling from the Maryland area)

International Bone Marrow Transplant Registry (IBMTR)/ Autologous Blood & Marrow Transplant Registry (ABMTR)
www.ibmtr.org
Medical College of Wisconsin
8701 Watertown Plank Road
P.O. Box 26509
Milwaukee, WI 53226
Phone: 414-456-8325
Fax: 414-456-6530
E-mail: *ibmtr@mew.edu*

International Cancer Alliance (ICARE)
www.icare.org/icare
4853 Cordell Avenue, Suite 11
Bethesda, MD 20814
Phone: 800-ICARE-61 or 301-654-7933
Fax: 201-654-8684

Iron Disorders Institute, Inc.
www.irondisorders.org
P.O. Box 2031
Greenville, SC 29602
Phone: 888-565-IRON (888-565-4766)

Iron Overload Diseases Association, Inc. (IOD)
www.ironoverload.org
433 Westwind Drive
North Palm Beach, FL 33408-5123
Phone: 561-840-8512

Leukemia & Lymphoma Society
www.lls. org
1311 Mamaroneck Avenue
White Plains, NY 10605
Phone: 914-949-5213
Toll-free: 800-955-4572
Fax: 914-949-6691

Myelodysplastic Syndromes (MDS) Foundation
www.mds-foundation.org
P.O. Box 353, 36 Front Street
Crosswicks, NJ 08515
Phone: 800-MDS-0839 (within US only)
609-298-6746 (outside US)
Fax: 609-298-0590

National Cancer Institute (NCI)
www.cancer.gov
NCI Public Information Office
Building 31, Room 10A31
31 Center Drive, MSC 2580
Bethesda, MD 20892-2580
Phone: 301-435-3848

Patient Registries at Slone: MDS
1010 Commonwealth Avenue
Boston, MA 02215
Toll-free: 800-231-3769
Fax: 617-738-5119
E-mail: *www.bu.edu/prs/mds*

Clinical Trials Information from the NCI
www.nci.nih.gov/clinical_trials

NCI-Designated Cancer Centers and Contact Information:
http://www3.cancer.gov/cancercenters/centerslist.html
National Comprehensive Cancer Network (NCCN)
www.nccn.org
Toll-free: 888-909-NCCN (888-909-6226)

National Hospice & Palliative Care Organization (NHPCO)
www.nhpco.org
1700 Diagonal Road, Suite 625
Alexandria, VA 22314
Phone: 703-837-1500
Fax: 703-837-1233
E-mail: *nhpco_info@nhpco.org*
Toll-free (English): 800-658-8898
Toll-free (Spanish): 877-658-8896

National Marrow Donor Program (NMDP)
www.marrow.org
3001 Broadway Street Northeast, Suite 500
Minneapolis, MN 55413-1753
Phone: 800-MARROW2 (800-627-7692)
Office of Patient Advocacy (OPA): 888-999-6743

Oncology Nursing Society (ONS)
www.ons.org
501 Holiday Drive
Pittsburgh, PA 15220
Phone: 412-921-7373

Patient Advocate Foundation (PAF)
www.patientadvocate.org
700 Thimble Shoals Blvd, Suite 200
Newport News, VA 23606
Toll-free: 800-532-5274

Social Security Administration (SSA)

www.ssa.gov
Office of Public Inquiries
Social Security Administration
Office of Public Inquiries
6401 Security Boulevard, Room 4-C-5 Annex
Baltimore, MD 21235-6401
Toll-free: 800-772-1213/800-325-0778 (TTY)

Veterans Health Administration (VHA)

www1.va.gov/health/index.asp
810 Vermont Avenue NW
Washington, DC 20420
Phone: 202-273-5400 (Washington, DC office)
Toll-free: 877-222-8387

Wellness Community

www.thewellnesscommunity.org
919 18th Street NW, Suite 54
Washington, DC 20006
Phone: 202-659-9709
Toll-free: 888-793-WELL
Fax: 202-659-9301

Well Spouse Association (WSA)

www.wellspouse.org
63 West Main Street, Suite H
Freehold, NJ 07728
Toll-free: 800-838-0879

Glossary

5q– syndrome: A subtype of MDS in which patients exhibit a specific chromosome abnormality characterized by loss of a portion of chromosome 5.

absolute neutrophil count (ANC): An estimation of the total number of neutrophils in the blood. The ANC is calculated by multiplying the total white blood cell (WBC) count times the percentage of neutrophils.

acetaminophen: A common pain medication used to treat pain. It is sold over the counter (Tylenol® and other brands) or as a prescription in combination with a narcotic for severe pain.

acute: Occurring within a short time frame.

acute myelogenous leukemia: A cancer affecting blood cells in which blasts reproduce rapidly but do not mature into normal white blood cells. This often occurs in conjunction with decreased red blood cells and platelets.

alkylators: A class of chemotherapy drugs that can sometimes lead to development of MDS or AML.

allogeneic: From outside the individual's body; used in reference to transplantation of cells from another person.

alloimmunization: The development of antibodies against red blood cells or platelets that can occur with repeated red blood cell or platelet transfusions, respectively. This can lead to difficulty finding compatible red blood cell units for transfusion or resistance to platelet transfusions.

anemia: A low red blood cell count.

aplastic anemia: A form of marrow failure caused by autoimmune attack on the marrow cells.

apoptosis: Cell death.

autoimmune: An immune response against the body's own tissues.

autologous: From within the individual's body; used in reference to transplantation of cells from oneself.

benign: Noncancerous.

blast: An immature white blood cell.

bone marrow: The central tissue of bones in which blood cells are formed.

bone marrow aspirate: Fluid bone marrow collected during a bone marrow biopsy.

bone marrow biopsy: Collection of bone marrow from a patient to determine presence of disease.

cellularity: The overall cellular composition of a tissue, such as bone marrow.

chemotherapy: Treatment involving the use of chemical agents, usually for cancer.

chromosome: Tightly wrapped chains of DNA. Each human cell has 46 chromosomes.

chromosome analysis: An examination of chromosomes in a cell to look for abnormalities, structural changes, or extra or missing chromosomes.

chromosome remission: A reduction or elimination of cells in which chromosome abnormalities are present.

chronic: Occurring over a long time frame.

circulation: The complete system of blood vessels that transports fluids, nutrients, and wastes in the body.

clonal: Referring to an abnormal cell that reproduces itself.

collagen: The principal protein within connective tissues. Its presence in the bone marrow is a marker of advanced fibrosis.

complete blood count (CBC): A laboratory test that counts the total quantity of blood cells in a blood sample.

core biopsy: Collection of solid bone marrow material by boring a cylindrical needle into the marrow for a sample.

cortex: Surface of the bone.

cytopenia(s): A low count of one or more blood cell types.

cytotoxic: Refers to substances, such as chemotherapy, that kill cells, particularly fast-growing cells.

deep venous thrombosis: A blood clot in a major vein, usually in the leg, that blocks the vein.

deletions: Refers to chromosomes that are missing portions of the genetic code present in normal cells.

differentiate: To cause an immature cell to develop into a mature cell.

DNA: Deoxyribonucleic acid, the molecule that forms the basis of all genetic information in human cells.

dysplasia: An abnormal, misshapen appearance.

erythroid precursors: Young, developing red blood cells found in the bone marrow.

erythropoeitin (EPO): A kidney hormone that stimulates red blood cell production in the bone marrow.

FAB classification: See French-American-British classification

fibrosis: Scarring of the bone marrow.

fluorescent in-situ hybridization (FISH): A type of chromosome analysis that can determine the presence of abnormal genes or chromosome segments.

French-American-British classification: A morphology-based MDS classification system published in 1982 by international investigators.

genes: Collections of DNA molecules that encode proteins that determine the basic structure and function of living cells.

genetic: Occurring within the genes.

genome: The complete sequence of human DNA.

graft-versus-host disease (GVHD): A condition in which cells within the donor infusion attack the recipient's cells.

graft-versus-leukemia (GVL): A phenomenon in which cells within the donor infusion attack the recipient's leukemic cells.

granule: A small particle within a cell that can be seen by light or electron microscopy; contains stored material.

granulocyte-colony stimulating factor (G-CSF): A hormone that stimulates white blood cell production.

granulocyte-macrophage colony stimulating factor (GM-CSF): A hormone that stimulates production of white blood cells, particularly macrophages.

hematocrit: The proportion of the blood volume that is occupied by red blood cells.

hematologist: A physician who studies blood diseases and disorders.

hematopoietic growth factors: Drugs that mimic certain blood proteins to stimulate the production of red or white cells in the bone marrow.

hematopoietic stem cells: Rare parent cells in the bone marrow that give rise to all blood cells.

hemoglobin: A molecule in red blood cells that is of key importance in transporting oxygen.

hemolysis: Destruction of red blood cells in the circulation.

histocompatibility: The extent to which a donor of blood or marrow matches the recipient's HLA type.

HLA-matched donor: An individual whose human leukocyte antigens (HLA) match those of a sick person such that a transplantation of healthy cells from the donor is feasible.

human leukocyte antigen (HLA): A system of genes encoding proteins that are unique to the individual. These proteins are used by the immune system to recognize native cells from foreign cells.

hypogranularity: A condition in which cells contain fewer granules than normal.

hypomethylating agents: A class of drugs that prevent methylation.

hypoproductive anemia: A form of anemia in which lowered production of red blood cells by the bone marrow is the cause of the low red blood cell count.

idiopathic: Of unknown origin.

Illinois needle: A needle with a syringe fitting for collecting fluid bone marrow.

immunosuppressive therapy: Treatment to suppress the immune system when autoimmune attack on the bone marrow is suspected.

incidence: A measure of new cases of a disease in a specific population during a particular time frame.

informed consent: Agreement by a patient to a medical procedure after having been carefully informed by the procedurist or hospital of what the purpose, risks, benefits, and nature of the procedure will be.

International Prognostic Scoring System (IPSS): A method of estimating risk of transformation to AML and overall survival for MDS patients

intravenous (IV) needle: A tube inserted into a vein to allow direct injection of medication.

investigational drug: A drug that has not received formal approval from the FDA for use in a particular disease.

iron chelator: A medication that removes excess iron from the blood.

iron overload: Excessive quantities of iron in the blood, which may lead to organ damage.

Jamshidi needle: A cylindrical needle with a cutting tip designed for collecting core biopsies.

leukemia: A cancer of the white blood cells.

leukocyte: Any type of white blood cell.

leukopenia: A low total white blood cell count.

lymphoid: Referring to the lymphatic system or lymphocytes—white blood cells that are a part of the lymphatic system and circulate in the blood.

malignant: Referring to cancerous cells that invade local tissue or tissue(s) outside the area of origin.

megakaryocytes: A developing cell in the bone marrow that gives rise to platelets in the blood.

methylation: A process in which tumor suppressor genes and other types of genes are inactivated by addition of a methyl group to the DNA. Deactivation of tumor suppressor genes can lead to growth of cancerous cells.

monocyte: A white blood cell that is responsible for consuming foreign substances in the body.

morphology: Shape or appearance.

multilineage dysplasia: Abnormalities of cell shape found in more than one cell line.

myeloablative: Referring to a treatment designed to kill off the patient's bone marrow cells prior to transplant.

myeloid: Any white blood cell that is not a lymphocyte (e.g., neutrophils, eosinophils).

myelosuppression: A reduction in blood cell counts due to a particular medication.

National Marrow Donor Program (NMDP) Registry: A national database containing HLA profiles of millions of potential donors.

neoplastic: Cancerous or having the potential to develop into cancer.

neutropenia: A low neutrophil count.

neutropenic fever: A fever occurring in a patient who has a low neutrophil or white cell count.

neutrophil: A mature myeloid white blood cell that is usually a first responder to bacterial or fungal infection.

non-steroidal anti-inflammatory drugs (NSAIDs): Drugs such as ibuprofen or naproxen used to treat pain, but that should be avoided in patients with MDS with thrombocytopenia because they inhibit platelets.

nucleus: The structure within a cell that contains the cell's genetic material.

nutritional deficiency: A condition in which intake of an important mineral, vitamin, or nutrient is insufficient for good health.

outpatient: Not requiring admission into a hospital or other healthcare facility.

pathologic: Indicative of disease or abnormality.

pathologist: A physician who examines blood, bone marrow, or other tissue samples to look for signs of disease or dysfunction in the cells.

performance status: A patient's overall health and ability to function.

peripheral venous access device: A catheter inserted into a peripheral vein for long-term drug therapy or blood monitoring.

pheresis: A method of collecting hematopoeitic stem cells or other cell types from the blood of a donor.

placebo: An inert substance that has no effect on body systems, used for comparison purposes in drug trials.

platelets: Blood cells that are important for clotting.

primary myelofibrosis: A disorder of the bone marrow sometimes confused with MDS with fibrosis.

procedurist/proceduralist: A person who performs a medical procedure and is responsible for describing the procedure to the patient and obtaining informed consent.

prognosis: Projected course of a disease in a particular patient based upon the factors in the individual's health history and in the nature of the disease itself.

prophylactic: A medication or treatment intended as a preventative for a likely complication.

pulmonary embolism: A blood clot in the lung.

radiation therapy: Treatment, usually for cancer, involving the use of radioactive substances to kill diseased cells.

red blood cells: Blood cells that transport oxygen from the lungs to the tissues.

refractory anemia with ringed sideroblasts (RARS): An MDS subtype characterized by the presence of ringed sideroblasts in the bone marrow.

reticulin: A type of structural fiber that crosslinks to form a fine meshwork, which acts as a supporting mesh in soft tissues such as liver, bone marrow, and the tissues and organs of the lymphatic system.

ringed sideroblasts: Red blood cells in the bone marrow that contain characteristic ring-shaped iron deposits.

secondary MDS: MDS that develops as a result of prior treatment with chemotherapy or radiation therapy for cancer.

Surveillance, Epidemiology, and End Results (SEER): A national database of cancer diagnoses that calculates the relative frequency of different cancers in the American population.

sequestration: Trapping of red blood cells in the spleen due to illness.

serum creatinine: A blood test that measures kidney function.

serum ferritin: A blood test which measures the amount of storage iron in the body.

serum sickness: Flu-like symptoms that are a side effect of horse or rabbit ATG.

stem cell transplantation: Transplantation of stem cells from another individual into a person with a bone marrow disorder or other disease.

subcutaneous: The fatty tissue underneath the skin.

supportive care: Care intended to improve quality of life without necessarily directly treating the disease.

symptomatic: Showing apparent effects of an illness or disorder.

syndrome: A collection of phenomena seen in association.

thrombocytopathy: A decrease in the ability of platelets to perform the clotting function.

thrombocytopenia: A low platelet count.

topoisomerase II inhibitors: A class of chemotherapy drugs that can sometimes lead to development of MDS or AML.

toxins: A poison; a substance that damages or harms a living organism or its cells.

transfusion reaction: A reaction in the patient who receives red blood cells or platelets. Transfusion reactions may have different causes.

trisomy: Presence of an extra copy of a particular chromosome.

tumor suppressor genes: Particular genes that prevent the development of cancerous cells.

umbilical cord blood: Blood samples collected from the umbilical cords of newborn babies that are stored for later use in stem cell transplantation.

unilineage dysplasia: Abnormalities of cell shape found in only one cell line, usually red blood cells.

white blood cells: Blood cells that fight infection, attack disease, mediate allergic responses, and heal damage to the body.

Index